Depressive Illness: Prediction of Course and Outcome

Edited by T. Helgason and R. J. Daly

In Collaboration with Other Members
of the EMRC Study Group on Mental Illness Research
E. E. Anttinen, H. Hippius, R. Sadoun and E. A. Sand

With a Foreword by H. Danielsson

Springer-Verlag
Berlin Heidelberg New York
London Paris Tokyo

Professor Tómas Helgason

Department of Psychiatry
National University Hospitals
101 Reykjavik, Iceland

Professor Robert J. Daly

Department of Psychiatry
Cork Regional Hospital
Wilton, Cork, Ireland

With 24 Figures and 20 Tables

ISBN-13:978-3-642-73548-6 e-ISBN-13:978-3-642-73546-2
DOI: 10.1007/978-3-642-73546-2

Library of Congress Cataloging in Publication Data. Depressive illness. Bibliography: p. Includes index. 1. Depression, Mental, 2. Affective disorders. I. Helgason, T. (Tómas), II. Daly, R.J. (Robert Joseph), 1936– . RC537.D455 1988 616.85'27 88-6659
ISBN-13:978-3-642-73548-6 (U.S.)

Softcover reprint of the hardcover 1st edition 1988

2125/3130-543210

ALLE ZEIT WACH
1842

European Science Foundation

This volume arises from the work of the Study Group on Mental Illness, a priority activity of the European Medical Research Councils (EMRC), which in turn is one of the five Standing Committees of the European Science Foundation (ESF). The EMRC, like the other ESF Committees, which cover the natural sciences, space science, humanities and the social sciences, brings together the research councils and academies of 18 European countries. Under the auspices of EMRC and ESF generally European scientists work on topics of common concern, co-ordinate the use of expensive facilities, and discover and define new endeavours that would benefit from a co-operative approach. Other typical work in the field studied in this book includes the European Training Programme in Brain and Behaviour Research, run by the ESF, closely linked with EMRC. In 1987 it brought together 500 young scientists from all over Europe in its Fellowships and residential courses.

Further information on EMRC and ESF activities can be obtained from:

European Science Foundation
1 Quai Lezay Marnésia
6700 Strasbourg, France

Foreword

The group of European Medical Research Councils (EMRC) was formed in 1971 and became a Standing Committee of the European Science Foundation (ESF) in 1975. EMRC is an association of medical research councils or equivalent organizations in Western Europe. The National Institutes of Health, the Israel Academy of Sciences and the European Office of WHO are associated with EMRC and take an active part in EMRC activities. The main aims of EMRC are to exchange information on the research policies pursued by its member organizations and to initiate and stimulate international cooperation in biomedical research. Since biomedical research is highly international in itself, EMRC concentrates its activities on furthering international collaboration in those fields where it can play a significant role as a complement to existing channels. Mental illness research has been judged by EMRC to fulfill these criteria.

After a survey of the activities of the member organizations in mental illness research, EMRC decided in 1978 to set up a study group to look for areas within this field to which EMRC could contribute. As a result of the work of the study group, four workshops have been arranged to define present knowledge in some specific areas and to delineate research needs. The present volume contains the proceedings of the fourth workshop, held in 1985 and dealing with the course and outcome of depressive illness. EMRC hopes that this volume will stimulate intensified research and research cooperation on mental illnesses.

HENRY DANIELSSON
Chairman of EMRC

Preface

Depressive illness is a common disorder with a variable course and outcome and excessive mortality, e.g., due to suicide. Although considerable progress has been made in the treatment of depressive illness over the past decades, many factors remain unknown making prediction of the course and outcome of depression difficult and calling for further research.

Selected papers presented at a workshop to identify needed areas of research in this field, organized by the European Medical Research Council's (EMRC) Study Group on Mental Illness Research in Cork, Ireland, in 1985 are assembled in this volume. To accomplish the purpose of the workshop, an attempt was made to bring together some expert opinions on different aspects of the course and outcome of depressive illness and to some extent of affective disorders in general without pretending to exhaust all aspects of the field. The important topic of treatment is not addressed specifically in this volume, although it was addressed at the meeting. Needed areas of research in the treatment of mental illness, including depressive illness, has been the topic of three previous workshops arranged by the study group, one on methodology in evaluation of psychiatric treatment (Helgason 1983), another on needed areas of research in the long-term treatment of functional psychosis (Helgason 1985), and the third on research strategies and design in psychological treatment of mental illness (Daly and Sand 1987).

The present volume contains two of the three major background papers prepared for the workshop with extensive review of the literature, i.e., the chapter on clinical course of affective disorders by Professor J. Angst and that on needed areas of research in the biological aspects of the prediction of course and outcome of depressive illness by Professor N. Matussek. The third background paper of the workshop, by Professor A. Jablensky, has already been published as an editorial in *Psychological Medicine* (1987).

Various other aspects relating to the course and outcome of depressive illness where further research is needed are discussed in different chapters. These range from genetic aspects to psychosocial aspects, from personality as a mediating variable in the pathogenesis of mood disorders, to physical ill health, age and depression, to brain imaging techniques in the study of depressive illness.

The publication of this volume could not have been realized without the cooperation and help of a number of people and institutions all of whom we want to acknowledge although only some can be mentioned here. The preparation of the workshop was undertaken by the members of the study group of mental illness research who are, in addition to the editors, Professors E. Anttinen (Finland), H. Hippius (Federal Republic of Germany), E. A. Sand (Belgium), and Dr. R. Sadoun (France) assisted by Dr. E. Schenk from the Secretariat of the European Science Foundation. The workshop as well as the research work presented there were supported by the member councils of the EMRC. Most of all our acknowledgement goes to the authors of the different chapters of the book as well as to other participants in the workshop. Last but not least we want to express our appreciation to the staff of Springer-Verlag for their patience, as well as the genuine interest and professional service given in connection with the publication.

Reykjavik and Cork 1988

TÓMAS HELGASON
ROBERT J. DALY

References

Daly R, Sand EA (eds) (1987) Psychological treatment of mental illness; research strategies and design. Springer, Heidelberg

Helgason T (ed) (1983) Methodology in evaluation of psychiatric treatment. Cambridge University Press, Cambridge

Helgason T (ed) (1985) The long-term treatment of functional psychosis; needed areas of research. Cambridge University Press, Cambridge

Jablensky A (1987) Prediction of the course and outcome of depression. Psychol Med 17:1–9

Contents

Contents

List of Contributors

You will find the address of each first mentioned author at the beginning of the respective contribution

Clinical Course of Affective Disorders

J. Angst

Introduction

Studies on the course of affective disorders have an impressive tradition that spans about 100 years. The classification has changed over these years and we can roughly distinguish three periods. The first begins with Falret's (1851) definition of bipolar disorders and the distinction between depression and bipolar illness. In 1889, Kraepelin unified all subgroups of affective disorders of patients suffering from either mania or depression, or both, and termed this the "manic-depressive psychosis." His influence dominated until the late 1960s when the papers of Leonhard et al. (1962), Angst (1966), Perris (1966), and Winokur and Clayton (1967) suggested a return to differentiating between monopolar, or unipolar, depression and bipolar disorder. Thus homogeneous subgroups such as mania or depression were mainly studied during the first of the aforesaid periods and during the past 20 years. The interest in studies on the course of affective disorders has greatly increased as a spin-off of the introduction of long-term medication and prophylaxis. From the therapeutic point of view, two questions arise: which patients should be selected for long-term medication, considering the relapse risk, and how long should such long-term medication be maintained, considering recurrence and the possibility of a burning out of the disorder in old age. Furthermore, the risks of long-term medication have to be weighed against the risks of nonrecovery or chronicity, social consequences of the disorder, and increased mortality or suicide.

Reviewing the literature on the course of affective disorders is difficult for a variety of reasons, such as the differences in methodology and patient sampling and the influence of treatment on the natural history of the disorder. Finally, only the synthesis of our entire knowledge on the course may allow inferences with regard to the untreated natural history. In this respect, studies that predate the introduction of ECT and psychopharmacological treatment are very relevant. Earlier reviews of the literature have been published by Weitbrecht (1949), Hastings (1958), Guze and Robins (1970), Winokur (1970), Achté (1973), Clayton (1978, 1981, 1983 b), Coryell and Winokur (1980, 1982), and Goodwin and Jamison (1984). The older monographs of the German literature will be taken into special consideration here (Mendel 1881; Emmingshaus 1887; Pilcz 1901; Rehm 1907; Saiz 1907).

Psychiatrische Universitätsklinik, PO Box 68, CH-8029 Zürich 8

From a methodological point of view, this review emphasizes the distinction between retrospective studies, follow-up studies, and prospective studies with repeated assessments. The selection of the patient samples studied requires particular attention. Our knowledge is severely biased by the fact that most of the studies are based on hospitalized patients, while only a small number deal with both outpatients and inpatients, and just a few are based on outpatients only. Practically no population surveys have been carried out.

Considering methodology, a number of interesting statistical approaches have been applied to longitudinal data of affective disorders. Life-table analysis has become widespread (Fleiss et al. 1976, 1978; Dunner et al. 1976; Dunn and Skuse 1981; Keller et al. 1982a, b, 1983; Lavori and Keller 1983; Lavori et al. 1984; Kovacs et al. 1984a, b). Dunn and Skuse have also applied Markov chain models and what they have called a "memory model" which takes the interaction between episodes into account. Period analysis has been used by Supprian (1973, 1975a–c, 1977) and autocorrelation analysis by Huba et al. (1976). Other procedures that have been applied are multivariate analysis or covariance (Tsuang et al. 1979), discriminant analysis (Murphy 1983), and multiple regression analysis (Angst and Weis 1967; Kay et al. 1969; Kerr et al. 1972; Johnson and Leeman 1977). This review concentrates as much as possible on the distinction of subgroups of affective disorders, mainly bipolar manic-depressive disorders and unipolar recurrent depression. In view of the fact that these two groups have many aspects of the course in common, they are usually discussed together.

The Ratio of Unipolar to Bipolar Affective Disorders

Court (1968) and Smeraldi et al. (1977) hypothesized a continuum of affective disorders, suggesting bipolar disorder to be a more severe form than depression. This hypothesis would make the mixed states more comprehensible (Court 1968). In this context, Bunney et al. (1972) suggested hypomania to be superimposed on depression, whereas Nunn (1979) suggested depression to be superimposed on hypomania. Independent of all theoretical concepts, recurrent unipolar depression and bipolar manic-depressive disorders can and should be distinguished on a phenomenological level.

The estimates of the ratio between unipolar and bipolar disorders depend on the definition of hypomania, the inclusion or exclusion of minor affective disorders, the type of sample studied (hospitalized patients or population surveys), and the method of classification (cross-sectional or longitudinal). A major source of error is underreporting of hypomania.

The estimates range widely: Boyd and Weissman (1981) estimated a ratio of 10–20:1. The Epidemiologic Catchment Areas (ECA) study has suggested a ratio of about 8 or 10:1 (Robins et al. 1984; Myers et al. 1984), while Krauthammer and Klerman (1979) estimated a ratio of 4:1, Bland and Orn (1982) 3:1, Kinkelin (1954) 2:1, and Egeland and Hostetter (1983) 1:1.

Angst et al. (1978) analyzed the change of diagnoses in hospitalized patients, using Bayes statistics. They concluded that an observed ratio of 8 : 1 for the first episode was in fact about 1 : 1 in view of the prospective follow-up and possible sources of error. This suggests that figures on the ratio of unipolar to bipolar affective disorder should be related to the length of observation. Cross-sectional surveys, even if based on lifetime prevalence estimates, cannot be conclusive.

Change of Diagnosis from Unipolar to Bipolar Disorder

The diagnostic stability of affective disorders was high in a blind 5-year follow-up study (Murphy et al. 1974a). A longitudinal diagnostic change from unipolar to bipolar disorder has been reported to a varying degree. As already mentioned, the rate of change depends on the length of observation and, in addition, it depends on the number of episodes experienced. Clayton (1981) summarized a wide range (4%–33%) of diagnostic change with an average of around 13%–15%. Earlier studies gave a rate of 4%–6% (Lundquist 1945; Winokur and Morrison 1973; Prien et al. 1974; Dunner et al. 1976). In a follow-up study over 34.5 years, Ciompi (1973) found 7% of diagnoses changed from unipolar to bipolar disorder. Perris (1966) reported a 13% change within a selected group of unipolar depressives who had experienced at least three depressive episodes. Higher rates were observed by Rao and Nammalvar (1977), with 39%. Brockington et al. (1982) observed in a 6-year prospective study a change in 29% of nonpsychotic major depressives (DSM-III), whereas such change occurred in 55% of cases of major depression with mood-congruent psychotic features.

Akiskal et al. (1983) noticed switches to hypomania in some outpatients even after 23–25 years. They found that in major depression DSM-III, followed on the average over 6.4 years, the "switchers" to bipolar illness had a significantly earlier age of onset (26 years) than the "nonswitchers" (35 years). In another study, Akiskal et al. (1978) followed 206 neurotic depressive inpatients and outpatients over 4 years; 22% of them had developed major depression as defined by DSM-III and 18% a bipolar disorder.

The switch can occur at any point of recurrence. While in the retrospective study by Johnson and Hunt (1979) all bipolars had switched from depression to mania after five episodes, this was not so in the study of Angst et al. (1978) where the switch occurred in many cases later, even after the tenth episode of so-called unipolar depressive illness. Angst et al. (1978) also found that the selection of patients with multiple depressive episodes does not homogenize a depressive group, but increases the switch rate and the probability of including bipolar patients. Shulman and Post (1980) described 67 elderly bipolar patients who had their first manic attack at about the age of 60 years.

A switch to hypomania has frequently been suspected to be drug-induced. The question has been dealt with extensively by Lewis and Winokur (1982) and by Angst (1985b). Both studies show that there is no clear evidence for such a phenomenon. A switch from depression to hypomania can also occur after withdrawal of tricyclic antidepressants and it has been suggested that this is a rebound phenomenon (Jones et al. 1984; Mirin et al. 1981).

Conclusion

The diagnostic stability of affective disorders in the longitudinal perspective is certainly high; a few percent of the cases become schizophrenic. But there is a considerable shift of diagnosis from unipolar depression to bipolar manic-depressive disorder, dependent on the length of observation. Therefore, the ratio of unipolar to bipolar disorder is usually overestimated.

Age of Onset

Data on age of onset are rather unreliable. The informants may not recall an early episode, or the illness can start with milder mood swings, minor depression, or hypomania which may (over the years) not be recognized as affective disorders. Such swings frequently occur during puberty – and years later, the patients may interpret them in retrospect as first episodes. The research by Kovacs et al. (1984a, b) illustrates this difficulty and shows that dysthymia in childhood or adolescence can be an early stage of primary affective disorder. In addition, the onset may be atypical in adolescence (Carlson et al. 1977). Akiskal et al. (1977) found in a follow-up study over 2–3 years that 35% of cyclothymics spontaneously developed a major affective disorder. This frequently unrecognized prodromal period may last over months, or years, and it can also occur in late-onset depressives (Hopkinson 1963). It can manifest itself with vague unspecific complaints and somatic symptoms.

There is no doubt that the distribution of observed ages of onset is affected by the underlying age structure of the population which is frequently not representative (Crowe and Smouse 1977; Heimbuch et al. 1980; Baron et al. 1983). It has been reported that age of onset may actually precede the first hospitalization by 10 years (Kinkelin 1954), and there is doubt whether it is adequate to use the criterion of an "initial consultation" as a measure of onset (Peselow et al. 1982). There is some indication that age of onset correlates between family members (Johnson and Leeman 1977) and that a positive family history of affective disorders is correlated with an earlier age of onset. The latter was found for manic-depressive disorders by Mendlewicz et al. (1972) and for unipolar illness by Hopkinson and Ley (1969). Angst (1966) found a higher morbid risk among first-degree relatives in patients with an earlier onset, whereas Johnson and Hunt (1979) could not confirm this finding. Age of onset does not differ in bipolar cases starting with mania or with depression (Johnson and Leeman 1977).

The statistical handling of data on age of onset is frequently unsatisfactory. Many authors describe age of onset by using the arithmetic mean. The distribution of the curve is heavily skewed to the left and the median is always lower than the arithmetic mean.

In addition, histograms of the distribution are rarely given, despite the fact that it may be bimodal or multimodal. This is of particular importance if unipolar and bipolar illness are taken together, as clearly illustrated by Slater (1938 b). But the same may also be true for bipolar psychosis. A bimodal distribution of age of onset can be a criterion for diagnostic heterogeneity, e.g., in the case of bipolar I and bipolar II disorders (Angst 1980 a). Some authors found a clear unimodal distribution in bipolar illness (Taylor and Abrams 1981; Loranger and Levine 1978). A unimodal distribution of age of onset of unipolar depressives was described by Peselow et al. (1982). But the figures are small and the age distribution is too narrow to be representative. A bimodal distribution may only show up if the patient population has a wide enough age span. A second peak is frequently created, for instance, by late-onset bipolar patients.

It has recently been shown by Baron et al. (1983) that the curve of the age of onset best fits a square-root normal function and that there is no difference between males and females.

As mentioned before, many studies give the mean age of onset. For bipolar disorders this is generally between 28 and 33 years (Wertham 1929 a; Clayton et al. 1965; Perris 1969; d'Elia and Perris 1969; Winokur et al. 1969; Baastrup et al. 1970; Woodruff et al. 1971; Carlson et al. 1974; Petterson 1977; Johnson and Hunt 1979; Glassner et al. 1979; Joyce 1984). Unipolar depression has definitely a later onset than bipolar illness. This has consistently been shown by all the studies, e.g., Kinkelin (1954), Angst (1966), Perris (1968), Woodruff et al. (1971), Angst et al. (1973 b), Taylor and Abrams (1973), Clancy et al. (1974), and Prien et al. (1974). While the median age of onset of bipolars is in the twenties, the median for unipolar depression is usually in the thirties (Berger 1909), or even in the forties (Nöthig et al. 1973).

A suspected sex difference (Nöthig et al. 1973) could not be confirmed for bipolar disorder (Wertham 1929 b; Perris 1968; Winokur 1975; Dunner et al. 1976; Johnson and Leeman 1977; Johnson and Hunt 1979; Joyce 1984). Only Perris (1966) found an earlier age of onset among bipolar males (25.5 years) than among females (35.2 years).

As mentioned above, the median is lower than the mean age of onset. This was illustrated, for instance, by Joyce (1984) who reported a median of 23 and a mean of 28 years. In a large study by Saiz (1907) the median age of onset of bipolars was under 20 years, that of manics between 20 and 24 years. There was no sex difference either. Loranger and Levine (1978) found a median of around 30 years for mania.

In face of the skewed distribution, some studies mention the percentage of an early onset at under 20 years of age. Rehm (1907) found this in 8% of manics, 7% of depressives, and 35% of manic-depressives. Most of the other studies show a considerably higher proportion of onset in adolescence, for instance, Mendel (1881) 19%, Wertham (1929a) 20%, Kraepelin (1921), and Winokur et al. (1969) one-third, while Baron et al. (1983) give 11%, Kinkelin (1954) 23.5%, and Rosen et al. (1983) 19% for bipolars. Baron et al. found 43% of bipolars with an age of onset under 30 years. An age of onset under 15 years is very rare. It was found in less than 1% of 2000 manics studied by Wertham (1929a). Recurrent depressives have an earlier age of onset than single-episode patients (Walker 1907; Umenhoff 1963).

An unsolved problem is single-episode and recurrent mania. These may be just variants of bipolar illness without depressive manifestation. But they have been described to have a later age of onset than bipolar illness (Taylor and Abrams 1973, 1981). Saiz (1907) found an age of onset under 20 in 22% of manics, and in about 50% of bipolar disorders.

Little research has been devoted to the subgroups of bipolar disorders as yet. Peselow et al. (1982) studied the age of onset defined as "initial consultation" in 90 patients with bipolar I, in 68 patients with bipolar II, and 96 with unipolar illness. They found a mean age of onset of 28 years, 31.5 years, and 35 years, respectively. Endicott et al. (1980) reported an age of onset of bipolar II patients at between 20.2 years for males and 21.8 years for females. Studies based on cross-sectional diagnoses of bipolar II disorder are not representative, because long-term follow-up studies show that a sizable number of so-called unipolar depressives may show hypomania in later episodes. Such cases are therefore not included if the patient sample is young and not followed long enough. Angst (1980a) broke down bipolar disorder into three subgroups, preponderantly manic (Md), preponderantly depressive (Dm, bipolar II), and patients with major mania and major depression (MD). The Md group had an age of onset of 32.6, the MD 31.6, and the Dm group 38.0 years. Thus, the two subgroups with major mania did not differ, whereas the bipolar II group showed a later onset. Peselow et al. (1982) described an earlier initial consultation for bipolar II patients with 29 years for females and 34.4 years for males. However, this difference might only reflect treatment-seeking behavior and not the age of onset.

Late age of onset is clearly correlated with more relapses (Swift 1907; Kraepelin 1921; Malzberg 1929; Paskind 1930; Pollock 1931b; Steen 1933; Lundquist 1945; Grof et al. 1974; Taschev and Roglev 1973; Zis et al. 1980; Angst 1980b; cf. section on cycle length). In a large study of a private practice, Watts (1956) described 529 depressives and found an earlier age of onset in reactive depression than in endogenous depression.

Cyclothymics have not yet been studied thoroughly enough. Akiskal et al. (1977) found an age of onset below 25 years in 60% of the cases.

Conclusion

Data on age of onset are unreliable and dependent on the age distribution of the sample studied. The hypothesis of a bimodal distribution of both unipolar and bipolar illness has not yet been investigated thoroughly enough. Bipolar disorder has definitely an earlier age of onset than unipolar depression. A sex difference is not present. Single-episode, and bipolar II cases may have a later age of onset.

Manic Onset of Bipolar Disorders

In his original material of manic-depressives ($n=899$), Kraepelin (1921) observed 471 cases at the first episode, of which 102 (22%) were manic, 106 (22%) biphasic, and 263 (56%) depressive. Some of the depressive cases may later have become bipolar; a follow-up was not given.

Many authors have analyzed the frequency of manic onset in bipolar illness, and the figures vary considerably from Rehm (1919) with 18%, to Dunner et al. (1976) with 79%. Rehm mentions another 39% with biphasic onset. Other authors give figures in between: Clayton et al. (1965) 26%, Perris (1968) 34%, Kinkelin (1954) 37%, Petterson (1977) 37%, Johnson and Hunt (1979) 40%, Lundquist (1945) 50%, Carlson et al. (1974) 50%, Winokur et al. (1969) 61%, and Landolt (1957) 78%.

Angst (1978) found that within bipolar illness, the ratio of manic to depressive syndromes remained stable over repeated episodes. But there was a remarkable sex difference, males having shown mania or both mania and depression in an average of two-thirds of episodes, whereas this was only so for 40% of the episodes in females. Purely manic syndromes were found in 35.3% of all episodes in males and 13.6% in females. Thus, within bipolar disorder, the females are more depression-prone. This finding could be an artifact, in that males would underreport depression or females underreport mania. The latter is however less probable. The question of biphasic or triphasic episodes has been dealt with by Winokur et al. (1969), who analyzed 100 manic episodes and found that 51% of them were preceded and 57% followed by depressive swings. More detailed figures of 95 patients and 1176 episodes were given by Angst (1978), distinguishing 12 different syndrome patterns of episodes, taking into account the severity and sequence of mania and depression, or of hypomania and mild depression.

Carlson et al. (1977) showed an equal age of onset of bipolar patients starting with mania or depression and thus could not confirm Perris's (1968) finding that males starting with mania would have an earlier age of onset. Johnson and Hunt (1979) described that patients with a positive family history of bipolar disorder were more likely to have a manic initial episode.

Investigations of unipolar mania are extremely rare. The most comprehensive early study was that of Saiz (1907) who reviewed the entire literature in his monograph and additionally analyzed 117 cases himself. He particularly concentrated on the question of simple mania, i.e., a single-episode disorder, which is known to be extremely rare and generally only diagnosed with a short observation period. Hinrichsen (1898) studied 233 manic patients at a Zurich hospital retrospectively and found only 17 of them (7.3%) to have remained relapse-free over 5 years. A similar report was given by Mayser (1899). Lambranzi and Perazzolo (1906) found seven of 320 manics (2.2%) to have remained relapse-free. The same was described by van Erp Taalmann Kip (1898) for only four of 856 patients (0.5%), two of which had been studied for only about 10 years. Vedrani (1905) found one manic case to have relapsed after 44 years. The results of all these investigations clearly demonstrate that simple mania cannot be considered a distinct entity.

Conclusion

A manic onset of bipolar disorders is probably more frequent in males than in females. Whether bipolar disorder starts with mania or depression has no prognostic value; age of onset is the same in both subgroups.

Number of Episodes

The observed number of episodes depends on many facts. Most of the studies are based on hospitalized patients who had usually experienced treated or untreated previous episodes. Therefore, figures on the percentage of single episodes vary to such a degree that they are almost useless. The number of episodes observed is of course a function of the length of observation since onset, which also varies from study to study (from 1 year to lifelong observation periods). Another variable is the definition of an episode. The number of observed episodes is also a function of chronicity. There are cases that become chronic right with the first episode. Finally, premature death or suicide also shortens the observation period. Several authors have tabulated percentage figures of single-episode courses in unipolar and bipolar illness, e.g., the reviews of Zis and Goodwin (1979), Coryell and Winokur (1982), and Bland and Orn (1982). For bipolar illness, the rates of single-episode cases vary from 0.5% to 55%, those for unipolar depression from a few to 61%. It is obvious that no conclusion can be drawn from these figures.

Some authors maintain that bipolar illness is definitely recurrent. Kinkelin (1954) reports 2.7% single-episode bipolar cases. Landolt (1957), who followed sixty 18-year-old bipolars over 5–25 years found only 10% with no recurrence. Fukuda et al. (1983) reported 8% bipolar illness with no recurrence. Murphy et al. (1974 b) reported relapses in all patients, but a relatively high rate of single-episode cases was recently given by Bland and Orn (1982) with 26%. On the whole, bipolar illness is usually recurrent, if observed over extended periods of time.

Unipolar depression may differ in this context. Angst and Frey (1976) found 19% single-episode cases in first hospitalized early-onset and 26% in late-onset unipolar depression. The higher rate in the late-onset group is due to a shorter observation period, shorter life, and higher chronicity. Our estimate is that unipolar depression is recurrent in about 70%–85% of all cases. The rates of nonrecurrent depression additionally depend on the diagnostic concept used. Including so-called reactive depression, the rates might be higher, and the same might be true for milder cases. But our population study shows that the recurrence of minor depression may be quite high (Angst et al. 1985).

There is no doubt that the total number of episodes observed is higher among bipolars than among unipolar depressives (Rehm 1907; Perris 1968; Bland and Orn 1982; Fukuda et al. 1983; Angst 1985a). The number of observed episodes is usually twice as high in bipolars as in unipolar depressives if the median is taken and the observation period is comparable (Bland and Orn 1982; Angst 1985a).

An interesting question is whether the episodes occur in bursts which are followed by quiescent periods, suggesting that no prediction of relapses is possible with any consistency (Coryell and Winokur 1982), and whether there is a "burning out" of the pathological process. The latter was found by Angst (1985a), following a large patient sample prospectively, in 29% of bipolar and 40% of unipolar illness at a median age of 66 years and 69 years, respectively. Burning out was defined as having been relapse-free over at least 5 years at the last follow-up.

An interesting fact is that unipolar mania might be less recurrent than bipolar disorder (Rehm 1907; Bland and Orn 1982). Unipolar mania is so rare, however, that this finding would be difficult to disconfirm. Furthermore, mania is even more underreported than depression. This is in particular true for hypomania which is frequently considered by the patient to be normal.

It has been proposed that affective disorders may have become more chronic (Till and Vuckovik 1970) or more recurrent due to the application of tricyclic antidepressants (Peley and Vargha 1974; Siris et al. 1979; Wehr and Goodwin 1979; Lerer et al. 1980; Tondo et al. 1981; Kukopoulos et al. 1983). In some cases there may be a true increase of episodes in a sense of "rapid cycling" (Siris et al. 1979) or, in others, just a fragmentation of longer episodes into briefer ones.

Conclusion

Single-episode mania seems to be extremely rare. The rates of single-episode depressive disorder vary considerably in the literature. They depend on the reliability of the data collected and the length of follow-up. Prospective studies collect more milder depressive episodes than do retrospective studies. Bipolar patients experience about twice as many episodes as unipolar depressives. In individual cases, an antidepressant treatment may induce rapid cycling. In general, the newer studies of inpatients and outpatients favor more and more a high recurrence of major and minor depression.

Length of Episodes

The length of episodes has been the subject of many investigations, most of which were carried out with insufficient methodology. Frequently, the arithmetic means are given which are not a suitable parameter for description. The distribution is a log-normal one, and logarithmic values or nonparametric parameters like medians and quartiles should therefore be used. Kraepelin (1913) gave lengths of 6–8 months and stressed that episodes can last only 8–14 days, but also a number of years. As an extraordinary observation, he mentioned the case of a patient who switched to mania after an 18-year-long episode of melancholia.

Studies predating the introduction of shock treatment and psychopharmacological treatment are of particular interest, because they reflect the spontaneous course much better than observations made during the last decades. Wertham (1929 a) collected data on 2000 manic attacks and computed an average duration of 242 days, but the majority was around 120 days. He also gave histograms which correspond very well to distributions later described by other authors (Angst et al. 1973 a). From Wertham's paper, we can extract that the median was between 120 and 180 days (4–6 months). In Mendel's monograph (1881) on mania ($n=43$) the median was between 5 and 6 months. In his textbook (1896), Ziehen estimated the length of an episode of depression to be 4–6 months. Pilcz (1901) gave a length of 3–6 months for manic and for depressive episodes in his monograph.

Huston and Locher (1948 a) gave a most detailed analysis of the duration of depressive episodes. They compared a control group of 63 patients with 65 patients treated by ECT. The control group had a median of 15 months, while the ECT group with 9 months definitely had shorter episodes. They tabulated the median of all depressive episodes as a function of the decade of onset. The 8 adolescents had a median of 3.5 months and the six patients aged 60–69 a median of 5 months, whereas the groups in between ranged from 7.5 to 9 months (total $n=196$). Analyzing depressive episodes with spontaneous recovery, the authors gave medians of between 3.5 months for adolescents and 6–8.5 months for depressives aged 30–59. Their figures illustrate very well how misleading mean values can be. The largest group, that of 30 to 39 year-old patients ($n=62$), had an arithmetic mean length of 14.8, but a median of 7.5 months.

Lundquist (1945) computed the median of recovered manic and recovered depressive patients, and he is the only one to have also given the quartiles Q1 and Q3. He found an increase of the median as a function of age. Patients younger than 30 years showed a median of 6.0 months for mania and 6.3 months for depression, whereas patients aged 50 or more had a median of 11.5 and 9.5 months respectively. These values are clearly higher than those of other studies. Matussek et al. (1965) analyzed 453 endogenous depressives and found a median of 4.5 months (males 5.0, females 4.0). The difference between the sexes disappeared if the first episodes were compared. Taschev (1965) found a median of 3 months for depressive episodes. Bratfos and Haug (1968) computed a median of 8 months for manic-depressive episodes, whereas the arithmetic mean was 13 months. Huhn and Pauly (1973) studied the manic episodes of 94 adolescents with bipolar disorder in a follow-up investigation. The median length of episodes was 4.6 months, 75% of the episodes lasted 6 months or less. More recently, Angst (1985 a) computed intraindividual medians over all episodes and found 4.2 months for bipolar disorder and 6.0 months for unipolar depression.

There is little doubt that the episodes of bipolar disorders are shorter than unipolar depressive ones (Swift 1907; MacDonald 1918; Rennie 1942; Lundquist 1945; Kinkelin 1954; Kielholz 1959; Bratfos and Haug 1968; Angst et al. 1973 a; Angst 1980 a). With higher age, the duration of episodes has also been reported to lengthen (Kraepelin 1921; MacDonald 1918; Wertham 1929 a, b; Pollock 1931 a, b; Lundquist 1945, Kawashima 1979), but this could as well be due to a minority of chronic cases. Another intervening variable is recurrence which was also postulated to produce a lengthening in some cases (Swift 1907; Pollock 1931 a, b; Rennie 1942), but the respective authors had not used multivariate models. Angst et al. (1973 b) could not confirm a lenthening with recurrence. Lundquist (1945) even reported that patients with repeated episodes had shorter periods.

Using life-table analysis, Keller et al. (1982 b) have shown that the recovery rate of major depressive episodes diagnosed using research diagnostic criteria (RDC) correlated with acuteness and severity.

In a prospective epidemiological study, Levinsohn et al. (unpublished) tabulated the length of three episodes separately. Unfortunately, the median was not given, but from two tables it can be estimated at 19–51 weeks, and from the third table (third most recent episode) at 18–19 weeks. There was no correlation with age of onset. These figures are important because they are more representative than those of hospitalized patients.

Conclusion

The length of episodes shows a log-normal distribution and should not be described by arithmetic means. Over this century, length of episodes has not changed clearly. Depressive episodes last longer than manic episodes (6 vs 4 months). There is no clear trend to an intraindividual change with recurrence.

Length of Intervals and Cycles

A cycle consists of an episode and the subsequent interval. The periodicity of affective disorders has usually been described by interval length. With psychopharmacological treatment this variable has become less reliable. The end of an episode is frequently blurred by the suppression of symptoms, while the episode may still be going on, which can be asserted by cessation of the antidepressant treatment. Therefore, and because the onset of an episode is easier to assess than its end, cycle length has more recently been taken as a more reliable variable.

In a remarkable study, Slater (1938 a) analyzed the length of intervals from a methodological point of view. He clearly showed that the analysis has to be carried out by breaking the patients down into subgroups. Lumping a whole sample together would engender the artifact of decreased cycle or interval length. Breaking the patients down by number of episodes, Slater gave mean values of interval length and showed that the first interval was definitely longer than the subsequent ones. The latter did not seem to show a definite trend. But faced with the skewed log-normal distribution and with the fact that the groups were very small, the reported arithmetic means are not representative. Swift (1907) had already estimated the length of the first interval to be $6^1/_4$ years and later intervals to be shorter. Rehm (1907) described the decrease in interval length to be present in depression and manic-depressive disorders alike. An irregularity of interval length with no systematic change has recently been reported by Cutler and Post (1982), as well as by Fukuda et al. (1983).

A decrease, at least after the first interval, has been found by numerous authors (MacDonald 1918; Lundquist 1945; Kinkelin 1954; Kielholz 1959; Angst et al. 1973 a; Zis et al. 1980). Kinkelin found a much longer first interval in unipolar depression, starting with 109.3 months, than in bipolar illness starting with 60.1 months, whereas, for instance, the 5th (25.7 and 24.1) and 6th intervals (14.4 and 12.1) were more or less equal.

There is wide agreement on the fact that a later age of onset correlates with shorter first and subsequent intervals (Swift 1907; Lundquist 1945; Kinkelin 1954; Angst and Weis 1967; Kawashima 1979; Zis et al. 1980).

A shorter interval and cycle length in bipolar illness as compared to unipolar depression is a well-established fact (Kinkelin 1954; Angst et al. 1973 b; Murphy et al. 1974 c; Angst 1980 a).

Some analyses have been devoted to the question of whether interval or cycle length depend on other factors, but multiple regression analysis (Angst and Weis 1967) has shown that only cycle number, age of onset, and age, are interfering variables. Whether so-called neurotic or abnormal disposition, or habitual, constitutional tendencies actually have any influence, as suspected by Swift (1907) and MacDonald (1918), is unknown.

The question whether cycle or interval length decrease or not, or whether there is at least a constant periodicity after the initial decrease in length is of practical importance. Several studies on prophylactic or long-term medication suggest that the past history predicts the frequency of future episodes, and it was generally assumed that there was no spontaneous decrease. This question has been a subject of some controversy, because "burnig out" is really possible in a number of cases. Angst (1984) found relapse-free burning out over 5 years in 29% of bipolars and 42% of unipolar depressives. Nevertheless, the majority of bipolar cases tend to be recurrent even into old age (Angst 1981).

Another interesting study is that of Kimura et al. (1984) who described 22 endogenous phasic psychoses in their course and prognosis. It is, however, not quite clear whether they were schizophreniform atypical psychoses or manic-depressive psychoses, some of them were probably schizoaffective. From a follow-up of 11 cases over 3–18 years (average 8 years and 9 months), the authors reported three suicides, a stable cycle length of 9.7 months, a mean length of episodes of 2.5 months, and no sex difference. The depressive episodes were shorter (1.6 months) than the manic (1.9 months) and biphasic episodes (3.7 months). The authors also described a lengthening of episodes and cycles in their follow-up, which is at variance with other papers.

Conclusion

The length of intervals or cycles should be analyzed separately for subclasses defined by the number of episodes. There is no doubt that the first cycle or interval is considerably longer than the subsequent ones. The question whether there is a log-normal decrease or a regular recurrence is controversial. Later age of onset correlates with shorter cycle length. Bipolar illness starts with shorter cycle length or intervals than unipolar depression.

Seasonality

Seasonal variations in affective disorders have lately gained attention. Seasonal depression or atypical depression has been reported to feature specific clinical traits and has become a subject of investigations regarding the application of light treatment (Rosenthal et al. 1984).

Seasonal variations in somatic and psychological disorders are frequent, and for affective disorders they had already been described by Aretaeus and by Hippocrates (according to Griesinger 1845; Zilborg 1941; Luce 1973). From a methodological point of view, one has to distinguish between studies that are devoted to the month of admission and studies that concentrate on the onset of episodes. A large investigation on the admission month was already carried out in 1897 by Mitchell who studied 3037 melancholics. He could not find any periodicity in the dates of admission. But by studying the onset of the episodes, he found a mild peak in April and December. The author stressed that not much variance was explained by the month of onset. In contrast to this result, Slater (1938 a) reported a clear peak of onset of manic-depressive episodes in May in 116 patients. A number of other studies found peaks of onset in spring or fall. The literature has been reviewed by Parker and Walter (1982) as well as by Rosenthal et al. (1983). There is some indication that bipolar populations may show two peaks of seasonal distribution (Angst et al. 1968; Rihmer 1980), whereas unipolar populations predominantly show one peak (Angst et al. 1968; Frangos et al. 1980). Mania seems to occur most frequently in spring and fall, according to Rosenthal et al. (1983).

In New South Wales, Parker and Walter (1982) analyzed the month of admission of 23000 patients with a depressive disorder and 3000 deaths due to suicide and self-inflicted injury over the years 1971–1976. They found a peak of admissions in spring for mania and reactive depressive psychosis, and a peak for depression in late winter. Male suicidal deaths did not show any significant seasonality.

Slater (1938a) pointed out that there may be an individual tendency to have seasonal onsets, which may not appear in analyses of total groups. Rosenthal et al. (1983) took an interesting approach by analyzing a single case over 13 years showing interesting regularities.

Conclusion

There are probably mild peaks of seasonal onset of affective episodes, but the explained variance is small. The phenomenon is probably overestimated. Further prospective single-case studies, and studies of subgroups are required.

Recovery

A review of the literature on the recovery from affective disorders is problematic. A variety of factors make studies comparable only to a certain degree: populations from hospitals, outpatient services, or even private practice; differences in diagnostics; differences in design (follow-up studies vs prospective studies); enormous differences in the length of follow-up period, which varies not only from study to study but also from patient to patient; varying definitions of "recovery." The figures given in tables 1 and 2 refer to studies which use the terms "social recovery," "not incapacitated," "well," "symptom-free," "good social adjustment," "complete remission," "return to earlier occupational level," "lasting recovery," "good outcome," etc.

We found about 29 communications, of which 11 refer to prospective, and 18 to follow-up studies. The follow-up studies have the advantage of covering much longer time periods than the prospective studies, but the disadvantage of not using repeated assessments. Most of the studies use all available sources of information, such as questionnaires or interviews of patients and/or other informants, records, etc.

The tables also list older studies, in order to give an estimate of whether and how the recovery rate has changed in the course of this century. Studies carried out in the first half of this century include those of Fuller (1935), Bond and Braceland (1937), Rennie (1942), and Lundquist (1945). These studies did not yet clearly distinguish between unipolar and bipolar disorder, except for Rennie's follow-up over 26–29 years (1942). But Rennie used a special criterion of "recovery of at least 5 years' length." It is nevertheless impressive that over 5 years, both his bipolar group ($n=49$) and his unipolar depressive group

Table 1. Follow-up studies – rates of recovery

Author	Year	Country	Sampling	I/O	Diagnosis	n	Follow-up (years)	Recovery %
Fuller	1935	USA				327	10	
Bond and Braceland	1937	USA	1927–1928	I	MDP	159	5	54
					ID	47		26
Rennie	1942	USA	1913–1916	I	M	17	26–29	35
					BP	49		29
					D	142		29
Lundquist	1945	Sweden	1912–1931	I	BP	103	8–27	85
					UP	216		76
Ziskind et al.	1945	USA	1938–1943	PP	D	109	1–5	75–88
Huston and Locher	1948	USA	1930–1939	I	ID	60	1–15	46
Watts	1956	UK	1946–1955	GP	ED	387	8	77
Hastings	1958	USA	1938–1944	I	M	42	6–12	40
					BP	26		40
					D+ID	112		47
Astrup et al.	1959	Norway	1938–1950	I	MDP	96	7–19	51
Post	1972	UK	1950	I	D>60	100	6	59
Shobe and Brion	1971	USA	1949–1953	O+I	M	5	18	47
					BP	10		
					<20	96		
Morrison et al.	1973	USA	1934/ 1944–1969	I	BP	87	35	51
					UP	59		61
Carlson et al.	1974	USA	1960–1970	I	BP	53	0.5–9	67
Winokur (Iowa 500)	1975	USA	1934–1944	I	BP	75	1–20	73
Tsuang et al.	1976	USA	1935–1944	I	BP	100	35	54
					UP	225		59
Rao and Nammalvar	1977	India	1974–1976	I	BP	36	3–13	77
					D	73		
Tsuang et al.	1979	USA	1934–1944	I	BP	86	30–40	50
					D	212		61
Zhenyi et al.	1980	China	1958–1978	I	AD	595	–20	67

Legend: See Table 3.

(n=142) showed a recovery rate of 29%, while the small manic group (n=17) recovered in 35% of the cases. Bond and Braceland (1937), in a follow-up over 5 years, found a recovery rate of 26% in 47 cases of involutional depression, which is definitely lower than that for their mixed group of manic-depressives (n=159) with 54%.

In face of the methodological differences between the various studies it makes more sense of compare the recovery rate of the diagnostic subgroups within the individual studies.

On the whole, the prospective studies cover observation periods ranging from 1 to 4 years, which is definitely not long enough to describe the course of affective disorders. In face of the short observation period, the higher recovery rates reported by some investigators may become understandable.

Table 2. Prospective studies – rates of recovery

Author	Year	Country	Sampling	I/O	Diagnosis	n	Follow-up (years)	Recovery %
Winokur et al.	1969	USA	1964–1965	I	M/BP	16	1.5–3	61
Post	1972	UK	1966–1967	O+I	D>60	92	1.5–3	63
Schapira et al.	1972	UK	1963–1965	I	D	28	(3.8)	46
Angst	1985	Switzerland	1959–1963	I	BP	105	17–21	23
					UP	139		42
Akiskal et al.	1978	USA		O+I	BP	18	3–4	86
					UP	22		
					SAD	10		
WHO	1979	International		I	D	72	2	39
					M	51		49
Klerman	1980	USA		O	ND	91	0.5; 1; 4	38–85
Keller and Shapiro	1981	USA		O+I	BP	15	1	93
					UP	86		71
Kovacs et al.	1981	USA		O	UP	35	1	46
Weissman et al.	1981	USA		O	D	62	1	48
Murphy	1983	UK	–81	O+I	D≧65	124	1	35

Legend: See Table 3.

Recovery rates largely depend on the length of follow-up and the definition of recovery, and they vary widely, which has mainly been shown by Winokur et al. (1969), Morrison et al. (1973), Tsuang et al. (1979), and Coryell and Winokur (1982). All these authors stressed the similarity in recovery between bipolar and unipolar affective disorders, a conclusion also drawn by Bland and Orn (1982). Some of the authors concluded differences in recovery rates between unipolars and bipolars, favoring the unipolars (e.g., Bratfos and Haug 1968; Shobe and Brion 1971; Morrison et al. 1973), whereas other authors stressed a better outcome for bipolars than unipolars (e.g., Lundquist 1945; Hastings 1958; Rao and Nammalvar 1977).

The hypothesis that bipolar and unipolar disorders do not differ to a significant degree is supported by several inpatient studies. Hastings (1958) followed 42 manics, 26 bipolars, and 112 depressives (including 53 involutional depressives) over 6–12 years and found a good adjustment in 40% of the manics and bipolars, and in 47% of the depressives. In the Iowa 500 study, 51% and 61% (Morrison et al. 1973) and 54% and 59% (Tsuang et al. 1976) of bipolars and unipolars, respectively, recovered. The WHO 2-year follow-up study of schizophrenia (1979) indicated a 49% recovery rate for manics and bipolars, and 39% for depressives. Thus, the few studies which covered unipolar and bipolar subgroups did not show considerable differences. The study by Keller and Shapiro (1981) does not include enough bipolars ($n=15$) to be conclusive.

Angst (1985a) found a difference between bipolar and unipolar illness in outcome if, in addition to social recovery, the criterion of a 5-year relapse-free follow-up was included. In such a case, bipolars were definitely worse, having only 23% recovery as compared to the unipolars with 42%. But this finding only reflects the bipolar group's higher proneness to further relapses.

More recently, an increasing number of studies have been devoted to outpatients (e.g., Klerman 1980), or a mixed group of outpatients and inpatients (e.g., Shobe and Brion 1971; Post 1972; Akiskal et al. 1978; Keller and Shapiro 1981; Murphy 1983). The recovery rates did not differ very much from those of inpatient studies. Unfortunately, the few studies including both subgroups did not differentiate between inpatients and outpatients in outcome, which would have been highly valuable.

A unique and thorough study of cases of endogenous depression ($n = 387$) in general practice with a follow-up period of 8 years was published by Watts (1956); he observed 77% recovery. In a prospective study of so-called neurotic depressives over 4 years Klerman (1980) found a relatively low complete remission rate of 38%, and it is remarkable that no deaths or suicides occurred.

A few studies have dealt with elderly patients (Bond and Braceland 1937; Hastings 1958; Post 1972; Murphy 1983), and it is of interest to note that one- to two-thirds of these patients showed a good recovery as reported for early-onset cases. Early- versus late-onset depressives did not differ in outcome in Murphy's study (1983). The remission rates given by Post (1972) covering follow-up periods in one sample over 6 years and another one over 3 years show an impressive 59% and 63% recovery (prospective study).

Keller and Shapiro (1981) reported on a retrospective 1-year follow-up study, breaking the affective patients down into unipolar and bipolar, primary and secondary, endogenous and nonendogenous, psychotic and nonpsychotic. Most of the differences were not significant, but this study is a good model for further research in this field, covering longer follow-up periods.

In sharp contrast to all those studies on affective disorders is the prognosis of bereavement. Bornstein et al. (1973) reported in a prospective study that after 1 year only 13% of the subjects were still depressed and after 4 years only one of 109 (Clayton 1980). This points to a major difference between bereavement and depression.

There is a lack of longitudinal studies of population samples, as already mentioned by Robins and Guze (1972). Hornstra and Klassen (1977) studied two community samples prospectively over 1 year, with a variety of instruments with weekly self-assessments and an interview after 12 months. Of 1171 adult Kansas City residents, aged 18 or more, 71% could be interviewed. The paper does not give recovery rates, but the authors pointed to the most striking finding that depressed mood persisted from year to year, and that enduring depression was not a temporary reaction to stressful life events.

In a field survey of two villages of West Bengal (India), Nandi et al. (1978) studied 2230 persons living in an agricultural area. After 1 year, spontaneous recovery was observed in 20 of 93 depressives (21.5%) only. Another study covering a population of 2020 persons from Oregon was carried out by Levinsohn et al. (unpublished), but comparable figures have not yet been published.

Conclusion

Recovery is not well defined and lies on a continuum from being symptom-free to suffering from mild or moderate symptoms compatible with social remission. The recovery rates depend on the length of follow-up. Therefore, the shorter prospective studies describe higher recovery rates than the longer follow-up studies. Recovery seems to be equal in both bipolar and unipolar affective disorders. Whether other diagnostic categories (primary-secondary, endogenous-nonendogenous, neurotic) are more predictive remains to be shown. Depression does not seem to have a worse outcome in the elderly. Further research in this area is needed. Up to now, there is no indication that outpatients might have a better outcome than inpatients. Figures about samples recruited from a normal population are not yet available.

Chronicity

The definition of chronicity is very difficult and varies from one author to another, as has been shown by Coryell and Winokur (1982). Frequently, "chronically disabled" is defined in a negative way, e.g., "not free of symptoms for any length of time" (Bratfos and Haug 1968) or "did not socially recover" (Lundquist 1945). In a more recent paper, Angst (1985a) used the criterion of the length of a nonremitting episode of 2 years, or more, for the definition of a chronic course. The difficulty consists in the distinction between an ongoing episode and a milder residual state during an interval. Up to now, there is no operational definition available to agree upon. The criterion used by Shobe and Brion (1971) "unable to work or to function socially most of the time," may be applicable. Despite a vague definition of chronicity, there is, however, an astonishing agreement about the frequency of a chronic outcome.

There is good agreement that chronic mania is a rare phenomenon (Barthomeuf 1888; Nitsche 1910; Wertham 1929b; Rennie 1942; Clayton 1983a). Following up first-onset manics, Lundquist (1945) found 8% chronic, Stenstedt (1952) only 4%.

The main source of variance between the authors is sample size. Coryell and Winokur (1982) mentioned 45% chronically disabled bipolar patients, published by Bratfos and Haug (1968), and 53% published by Shobe and Brion (1971). Poort (1945) reported a 56% chronicity rate. All these papers were based on less than 20 cases for which reason these figures should obviously no longer be quoted in reviews of the literature. Most other studies, with sizable patient samples, found a chronicity rate between 10% and 25% in both unipolar and bipolar disorder.

The rate of chronic affective patients does not seem to have changed considerably during this century. While Rehm (1907) reported 7% for depression and 29% for bipolar disorders, Berger (1909) found 10%–17% chronicity in early- and late-onset cases of unipolar patients, figures which do not differ from recent publications. Clayton (1981) estimated that about one-third of bipolar patients may have a chronic course, but many authors reported lower figures based on large samples, e.g., Rennie (1942) 11%, Lundquist (1945) 8%, Stenstedt (1952) 4%, Winokur et al. (1969) 11%, Carlson et al. (1974) 12%, Morrison et al. (1973; Iowa 500 study) 21%, Kinkelin (1954) 39% (small sample, $n = 57$).

Ciompi (1973) found 20% chronicity for unipolar depression in a long-term outcome study. Kinkelin (1954) found 14% and Bratfos and Haug (1968) 23%, whereas from the Iowa 500 study, Morrison et al. (1973) reported 20%.

The statement by some authors that chronicity was more frequent among bipolars than unipolars is not based on large enough samples, e.g., Poort (1945), Kinkelin (1954), Bratfos and Haug (1968), Shobe and Brion (1971). Lundquist (1945) found the opposite to be true, based on a larger material. In our prospective study over 15–20 years (Angst 1985 a) we found chronicity, defined as nonrecovery for over 2 years or more from the last episode, in 14% of unipolar depression and in 12% of bipolar disorders.

Other subgroups of affective disorder have rarely been studied. Reviewing the literature, Carlson et al. (1977) came to the conclusion that about one-fourth of adolescents with affective disorders may develop chronicity. Endogenous depression may more frequently result in a chronic outcome than reactive depression, as stated by Forssman and Jansson (1960) and by Refsum and Astrup (1980), where the diagnoses were made blindly.

Table 3 shows that most of the studies on course referred to here are based on hospitalized patients. An exception is the paper of Berti Ceroni et al. (1984) who reported an extremely high rate of chronicity (20 of 26 ambulatory cases), but the greater part of the sample was not followed up sufficiently long ($n = 111$). In Shobe and Brion's (1971) paper, there may be about 50% ambulatory patients; the depressed group is sizable enough to draw conclusions, 14.6% did not recover. This figure is within the range of the studies of hospitalized patients. In outpatient treatment studies, the rate was between 20% and 25% (e.g., Kovacs et al. 1981; Weissman et al. 1981).

An interesting exception is the epidemiological study of Schipkowensky and Milenkow (1970) based on all patients registered in a given geographic area of Bulgaria (outpatients and inpatients). During the follow-up period of 10–15 years, 11.9% developed chronicity. Unfortunately, the material was not differentiated into subgroups of manic-depressive disorders.

The long-term observation of so-called chronic cases is very interesting and important. Wertham (1929 a) observed recovery in mania after a so-called chronic course of 5–11 years length; Winokur and Morrison (1973) and Morrison et al. (1973) also stated that chronicity may have a limited life of up to about 10 years. A large number of such cases with a late recovery were described by Kreuser (1900).

A number of studies analyze factors correlating with chronicity, such as diagnosis, age of onset, age, coexistence with physical illness, psychopathology

Table 3. Chronic outcome

Author	Year	Country	I/O	Diagnosis	n	Design (years)	Chronicity %
Mendel	1881	Germany	I	M	57		20
Berger	1909	Germany	I	D	238	R 12	12.6
Rehm	1919	Germany	I	MDP	400	R	8
Kraepelin	1921	Germany	I	MDP	899	F 10–40	4–5
Mauz	1930	Germany	I	MDP	420	F	10
Bond and Braceland	1937	USA	I	MDP	159	F 5	19
				ID	45		22
Rennie	1942	USA	I	UP	142	F 26–29	13.4
				BP	55		10.9
				UM	16		6.2
Lundquist	1945	Sweden	I	MDP	319	F 30	
				M	103		8
				D	216		26
Poort	1945		I		<20	F 10–15	33
Huston and Locher	1948	USA		ID	60	F 1–15	18
				UP	80	F 7	9
Kinkelin	1954	Switzerland	I	UP	89	R 1–27	14.6
				BP	51		41
				UM	6		16.1
Watts	1956	UK	GP	ED	387	F 8	14
Landolt	1957		I	BP	44	F 5–25	16
Hastings	1958	USA	I	D	67	F 6–12	31
				M	42		27
				BP	26		27
Astrup et al.	1959	Norway	I	MDP	96	F 7–19	19.8
Forssman and Jansson	1960	Sweden	I	ED	97	F 5–10	24
				RD	99		8
Bratfos and Haug	1968	USA	I	MDP	207	F 6	23
Winokur et al.	1969	USA	I	M/BP	28	P 1.5–3	11
Schipkowensky and Milenkow	1970	Bulgaria	E	MDP	821	R 10–15	11.9
Shobe and Brion	1971	USA	I+O	D	96	F 14–20	14.6
				M	5		40
Post	1972	UK	I+O	ID	81	P 6	17.1
				ID	92	3	11.9
Schapira et al.	1972	USA	I	D	28	P 3.8	10.7
Ciompi	1973	Switzerland	I	D	127	F 20.5	20
				M	28	34.5	
Winokur and Morrison	1973	USA	I	UP	108	F 10–20	1
Carlson et al.	1974	USA	I	BP	49	F 0.5–9	12
Carlson et al.	1977	USA	I	BP	28	F 0.5–9	20
Rao and Nammalvar	1977	India	I	BP	36	F 3–13	8
				D	73		11
Akiskal et al.	1978	USA	O	PD	40	P 3–4	10
WHO	1979	International		D	72	P 2	7
				M	51		2
Klerman	1980	USA	O	ND	91	P 0.5; 1; 4	25
Kovacs et al.	1981	USA	I	D	35	P 1	26

Table 3 (continued)

Author	Year	Country	I/O	Diagnosis	*n*	Design (years)	Chronicity %
Coryell et al.	1983	USA	I	UP	44	F 5	18
Murphy	1983	USA	O	D	124	P 1	29
Berti Ceroni et al.	1984	Italy	O	D	111	P 1–4	77
				BP	9		44
Angst	1985	Switzerland	I	UP	139	P 15–20	14
				BP	105		12

Legend: *I*, inpatients; *O*, outpatients; *GP*, general practice; *E*, epidemiological study; *PP*, private practice; *M*, mania; *D*, depression; *MDP*, manic-depressive psychosis; *ID*, involutional depression; *UP*, unipolar depression; *BP*, bipolar illness; *UM*,unipolar mania; *ED*, endogenous depression; *RD*, reactive depression; *PD*, primary depression; *ND*, neurotic depression; *AD*, atypical depression; *R*, retrospective study; *F*, follow-up study; *P*, prospective study.

(delusions, hallucinations), presence of adversive life events, personality, number of previous episodes, etc. There is no agreement about the effect of age of onset or age. While MacDonald (1918) and Lundquist (1945) found a higher age being correlated with a chronic outcome in unipolar depression, Winokur and Morrison (1973) could not confirm this, nor could they find a correlation with age of onset. Among 821 cases of manic-depressive psychoses (without breakdown into depression or bipolar disorder), Schipkowensky and Milenkow (1970) found 12% chronicity and an increase with age, as it was also reported by Rao and Nammalvar (1977) for the age group over 40.

Milenkov and Apostolov (1969) found an increase in chronicity with higher number of episodes, which was also described by Bratfos and Haug (1968). A sex difference in chronicity was not found by Schipkowensky and Milenkow (1970), but women showed more chronicity in the Iowa 500 study (Winokur and Morrison 1973; Morrison et al. 1973). The presence of senile dementia was not found to be elevated in depressed elderly peoply (Murphy 1983), but there is good evidence that poor outcome in elderly people is partly due to a higher frequency of delusions and hallucinations and mainly to the presence of physical illnesses (Roth and Kay 1956; Post 1962, 1972; Kay and Bergmann 1966; Cole and Hicking 1976; Murphy 1983). Murphy (1983) hypothesized that physical illness may have an unfavorable effect by the psychological meaning of such an unfavorable life event. This conclusion was based on the assessment of life events using the method of Brown and Harris (1978).

Poor outcome in elderly people is frequently linked with acute or chronic physical illness and physical symptoms, or disorders, which are sometimes overlooked and diagnosed as hypochondriasis (Roth and Kay 1956). Physical illness is particularly frequent in males. Roth and Kay do not support the assumption of a symptomatic or secondary depression in most of the cases. The physical and psychiatric disorders did not pursue a parallel course, e.g., depression recovered but physical illness continued, or the opposite occurred. Elderly depressives with minor organic signs had a poorer prognosis and were less likely to be discharged from hospital, as reported from the 2-year follow-up investigation carried out by Cole and Hicking (1976). The issue of concurrent physical disorders is dealt with in more detail in the section on mortality.

Akiskal (1982) enumerated a variety of environmental factors correlating with chronicity, e.g., multiple losses through deaths of family members, disabled spouses, concurrent incapacitating medical diseases, and secondary abuse of drugs or alcohol. He also found chronicity significantly correlated with a positive family history of affective disorders.

Conclusion

Chronicity defined as nonremitting episodes over 2 years, or more, may be present in 10%–20% of patients suffering from affective disorder. Bipolar and unipolar subgroups do not differ. In following the patients long enough, chronicity may get a limited life; chronic episodes may resolve after many years. Chronicity is correlated with many factors, particularly with chronic physical illness in elderly patients.

Residual Symptoms

Not all affective episodes remit completely. The course is frequently worse than expected (Kinkelin 1954). Pilcz (1901) discussed the effect of hospitalization inducing changes of the temperament in the sense of becoming irritable, unpredictable, indolent, and egocentric. Meyer (1874) described a lowered reactivity as a residual phenomenon. Von Hösslin (1909) studied late-onset manic-depressive psychoses at the beginning of this century, and extensively described patients being in the hospital with a loss of interest, loss of reactivity to visits of relatives, and egocentric, apathetic, and dumb behavior.

A great number of residual symptoms have been described by German psychopathologists, such as neurasthenia (Stransky 1911), loss of potential (Conrad 1958), dynamic loss (Janzarik 1959), pure defect (Huber 1966), exhaustion, depressive reaction, low efficiency (Buerger-Prinz 1961; Weitbrecht 1967), loss of drive, exhaustion, low stress tolerance, emotional instability (Lauter 1969; Glatzel and Lungershausen 1970).

A review of intermediate outcome was given by Cassano et al. (1983).

Ciompi (1973) found longitudinally with increasing age a flattening of episodes and the development of a chronic residual state characterized by being weak, tired, hypochondriacal, dysphoric, discontent, irritable, distrustful, and anxious. The residual states seem to be more frequent among bipolars than unipolars which was also mentioned by Lauter (1969). Weitbrecht (1961) described loss of vitality, a dynamic loss, and sleep deficits as residual symptoms of depressives, and egocentric, irritiable, almost hypomanic, overactive, and disinhibited behavior in early-onset manics.

An exception is the study of MacVane et al. (1978) who compared 35 remitted bipolar patients with 55 controls and could not find any differences using several instruments for the assessment of residual symptoms or personality.

Conclusion

The assessment of residual symptoms has not yet been conducted systematically enough. The knowledge in this field is still very scarce.

Time Spent in Illness, Social Consequences

Oltman and Friedman (1962) studied the life cycles of 187 manic-depressive patients. The 84 males spent 38% and the 103 females 34% of their lifetime after onset of the disorder in hospital. Brockington et al. (1982) studied unipolar depressives prospectively over 6 years and found that the nonpsychotic group spent 17.1% and the mood congruent psychotic group 15.3% in hospital. Coryell and Norten (1980) compared adolescents, studied on the average over 5.7 years, and adults, studied over 8.4 years. Time spent in hospital was 12.6% and 9.4%, respectively. Breitenmoser (1971) found that in Zurich, the hospitalization rates of depressives were on the average 29% longer prior to the introduction of psychotropic drugs. Precipitated episodes of major depression stayed on the average 13% longer in hospital, and single people spent 40% more time in hospital than married people.

In the prospective Zurich study (Angst 1985a), the computed time spent in illness (episodes) after the onset of the disorder over an average observation period of 26 and 19 years was 20% in bipolar depression and 23% in unipolar depression, suggesting no difference between the two groups.

In face of the recurrent course and the fact that not all episodes remit completely, a great number of social consequences have been described. According to Tsuang et al. (1979), studying the Iowa 500 sample, the consequences are the same in bipolar and unipolar disorder. They consist in marital, residential, and occupational problems as well as psychiatric symptoms. Clayton (1984) described school, job, and marital disruptions and, in addition, alcohol abuse. The loss of productive time over 14 years was estimated at 11.4% in bipolar, 15.9% in unipolar depression, and only 2.8% in single-episode depressives, whereas for schizophrenics, it was 28% (Tsuang et al. 1979).

Conclusion

After onset of the illness, about 20% of the lifetime remaining is spent in episodes. There is no difference between bipolar and unipolar disorders. A great number of social consequences have been described. They are especially severe in early-onset cases and consist in marital, residential, and occupational problems.

Mortality

There is an increased mortality rate in affective disorders. Death can occur during an index episode, during subsequent episodes, or in the intervals. However, these three aspects have not yet been separated well enough. Pollock (1931 a) reported 9% (756/8438) deaths among first admissions for manic-depressive disorder in New York State, covering the 1909–1920 period. An even higher figure was given by Derby (1933) for the time-period 1912–1932 with 22.5% deaths (980/4341) among admissions for manic-depressive disorder. A much lower rate was reported by Poort (1945) for the time period 1928–1932 in Denmark with 4.4% (11/250). There is no doubt that the rates are considerably lower today and more frequently due to suicide, whereas in earlier decades more physical disorders and exhaustion during manic episodes had increased the death rate. Modern treatments decrease the death rate of manic patients (Tsuang and Winokur 1974). ECT reduces the death rate of unipolar depressed patients (Huston and Locher 1948 b; Avery and Winokur 1976) and this effect is not only due to reduction of suicide (Ziskind et al. 1945), but also of mortality in general (Huston and Locher 1948 b). The elevated mortality was most convincingly shown again with the Iowa 500 study (Tsuang and Winokur 1974; Tsuang and Woolson 1978; Tsuang et al. 1979, 1980 a, b).

As compared to the normal population, the mortality of the unipolar depressives is elevated (Stenstedt 1959; Kay and Bergmann 1966; Evans et al. 1974; Ciompi and Medvecka 1976; Tsuang and Woolson 1978; Tsuang et al. 1979, 1980 a; Baldwin 1980; Fukuda et al. 1983; Murphy 1983), as is that of patients with bipolar disorders (Perris 1966; Tsuang et al. 1980 a; Clayton 1984). The mortality of patients with bipolar disorders was, in a 50- to 60-year follow-up study clearly increased (Petterson 1977), and Perris (1966) found a higher mortality among bipolars than among unipolar depressives. The authors agree that the mortality is especially elevated in the depressed elderly (Stenstedt 1959; Kay and Bergmann 1966; Post 1972; Jacoby 1981; Evans and Whitlock 1983). A sex difference in mortality was not found by Fukuda et al. (1983), but was found by Tsuang et al. (1980 a).

The increase in mortality is most pronounced in the first decade (Derby 1933; Tsuang and Woolson 1977; Tsuang et al. 1980 b), and this is due to the distribution of suicides (Guze and Robins 1970). In elderly patients of age 40 and more, the mortality of early- and late-onset cases is the same according to a 4-year follow-up study by Evans and Whitlock (1983).

The higher mortality is not only due to the high rate of suicide, but also to physical diseases in general. A suggested high prevalence of carcinoma (Kerr et al. 1969) was not corroborated by Evans et al. (1974), Baldwin (1980), or Tsuang et al. (1980a, b). There is good evidence that the following diseases may occur rather frequently: diseases of the circulatory (Tsuang et al. 1979) and respiratory system (Evans and Whitlock 1983), arteriosclerotic heart disease and vascular lesions of the CNS (Rehm 1919; Baldwin 1980), cerebral vascular disease (Kay 1962), diabetes mellitus in bipolar illness (Rehm 1919; Lilliker 1980), and atopic disorder (Nasr et al. 1981).

Based on 1489 persons with affective psychoses and 3915 nonpsychotic depressives, the Oxford record linkage study by Baldwin (1980) gives convincing data on the association of physical disorders with affective psychosis and with depression. The risk for cancer is not elevated, but the risk for arterioslerotic heart disease and vascular lesions of the CNS is. Among depressives there is an increased risk for hypertensive heart disease, other hypertensive disease, and arteriosclerosis in general. There is also an elevated risk for pneumonia and bronchitis and, in depression, for pulmonary tuberculosis. Furthermore, the risk for asthma, hay fever, peptic ulcer, diabetes mellitus, thyreotoxicosis, and myxoedema is elevated.

Conclusion

Patients with affective disorders have an increased mortality, on the one hand due to suicide and on the other hand due to a higher morbidity for physical diseases. There is good evidence for a higher risk of arteriosclerotic and vascular disorders in the periphery and in the CNS, probably also for atopic disorder and diabetes mellitus, for infectious disease, and for thyroid dysfunction.

Suicide

Worldwide, suicide tends to be underreported, and some cases are concealed within the group of "accidental deaths" (Tsuang and Woolson 1978). A general review of the epidemiology and risk factors of suicide has recently been published by Clayton (1983b). Suicide rates of affective disorders in follow-up studies can refer to all deaths observed or to all patients observed. Usually, the former figures are given, as, for instance, in the well-known review of Guze and Robins (1970). In 9 of 17 studies they found a suicide rate of 12% to 19% of all deaths. The other studies showed still higher suicide rates. Of course, both figures – those of suicides and those of all deaths – depend on the length of the follow-up period, which is rather short in most of the studies. The ideal information would consist in suicide rates gathered from a total sample studied over lifetime. Analyzing length of follow-up and suicide rate together, Guze and Robins came to the conclusion that about 15% of the deaths were due to suicide. Coryell and Winokur (1982) found that the risk of suicide was greater in males and increased with age. The suicides usually occur at an early stage of the illness, mainly within the first 10 years (Guze and Robins 1970; Clayton 1983b; Tsuang and Woolson 1978). In a 3-year prospective follow-up study (Lönnqvist et al. 1983) of hospitalized psychiatric patients, the risk for natural death was 2.3 times elevated in affective psychoses and 2.5 times in manic depressives. The risk for suicide was about 30 times that of a normal population. In the prospective Lundby study by Hagnell et al. (1981) the suicide rate of male depressives was 13 times higher than expected.

The suicides show a small peak in spring (Taschev and Roglev 1973). Patients who committed suicide had usually communicated their intent during their lifetime (Fowler et al. 1979).

An interesting question is whether there is any difference between suicide rates in unipolar depression and bipolar disorder. Taschev and Roglev (1973) reported a suicide rate of 18.8% in involutional melancholia, 32.4% in recurrent depression, and 33.3% in bipolar disorder. Tsuang and Woolson (1978) found 9.3% for manics and 8.0% for depressives. Tsuang reported from the Iowa 500 study a rate of 9.3% for unipolar depression and 11.1% for bipolar disorder, versus 1.9% for the controls. Perris (1966) reported a higher rate in his unipolar depressives with 27% (20/75) than in his bipolar patients with 11% (3/27), which is close to Tsuang and Woolson's (1978) figures of 11.5% (6/59). Angst (1980a) found in a prospective study over 19–26 years a suicide rate of 24% among unipolar and 9% among bipolar disorder. A low suicide rate among bipolars was also found by Petterson (1977) with 5%. The hypothesis that the suicide rate may be lower among bipolar disorders should be the subject of further investigation. Up to now, there is not enough evidence to assume a difference.

Rates of suicide attempts may be more or less the same in bipolar disorders (26.1%) and in unipolar depression (20.9%), as reported by d'Elia and Perris (1969). Repeated suicide attempts were observed in 26% of the patients, and their distribution over episodes was irregular. Suicide attempters and contemplators were distributed more or less equally over bipolar I, bipolar II, and unipolar affective disorder among patients from a lithium clinic ($n = 205$) as reported by Stallone et al. (1980). Fowler et al. (1979) reported from the Iowa 500 study that suicide attempters showed a higher rate of subsequent relapses.

Conclusion

Suicide tends to be underreported, and up to now there has been no indication for a reduction of the risk during this century. Suicide is still a frequent outcome, estimated to be within the range of 10%–15% of affective disorders. Neither suicides nor suicide attempts seem to be different in bipolar disorder or unipolar depression.

Prediction

Analyses of predictive factors of the course are difficult to carry out. Sex has been studied widely, and it has been suggested that males would have a better outcome (Astrup et al. 1959; Kerr et al. 1972). Bratfos and Haug (1968) found a lower relapse rate in men, but more chronicity in the age group over 50 in a follow-up study over 6 years.

Astrup et al. (1959) found a better outcome if the patient had an acute onset and few attacks, Kerr et al. (1972) if the age of onset was high and the duration of the attack brief, whereas psychological precipitation and early life events did not have any influence. The prognosis was worse if neurotic or phobic symptoms were present in childhood, if the personality showed hysterical traits, and if there was marital disharmony. Nuller et al. (1972) agree with the fact that peculiar personality traits correlate with a more doubtful prognosis.

Kay et al. (1969) found a better prognosis in endogenous retarded than in neurotic depressives with somatic complaints. The same, measured by readmissions to hospitals, was found by Saran (1971) for reactive depressives as compared to endogenous cases. This agrees well with Paykel et al.'s (1974) finding that neurotic depressives were worse in outcome than endogenous depressives. Weissman et al. (1978) studied 150 neurotic depressive female outpatients over 4 years and found the neuroticism score measured by the MPI to be predictive, but not the initial severity of depression. Keller et al. (1982a) distinguished between prediction of recovery, which correlates with acuteness of the onset and severity of the illness, and prediction of relapses which is dependent on the length of a free interval and the number of previous episodes. Lundquist (1945) mentioned that length of illness prior to treatment was predictive. In patients with an ill spouse due to assortative mating, Merikangas et al. (1983) found in a follow-up over 1–3 years a poorer social adjustment, but no difference in relapse rates. A family history of mental illness did not predict relapse rates either (Landolt 1957; Gangil et al. 1982). Secondary depression and higher age of onset clearly correlate with a likelihood of relapse, as shown by Keller et al. (1983) using life-table statistics, and by Angst and Weis (1967) using multiple regression analysis.

A higher relapse risk was found in children and adolescents by Kovacs et al. (1984b) in the presence of double depression (Keller and Shapiro 1982).

Conclusion

The data on prediction of the course and outcome are inconclusive and probably in their majority sample-dependent. Further research in this area is badly needed.

Affective Disorders in Childhood and Adolescence

Melancholia and bipolar affective disorders have been well known throughout the nineteenth century, but were considered to be rare in childhood. Already in the middle of the last century, Berkhan (1863) gave a large review of the literature which goes back to the eighteenth century. He described the case of a 6-year-old boy with delusional melancholia, with an onset at age 5 and later episodes with complete remission in puberty. Steiner (1873) mentioned a 6-year-old boy with a 2-year hypochondriacal melancholic episode. Zeller (1844), one of the leading psychiatrists of the last century, described a 9-year-old with manic-depressive disorder and mentioned cases with an age of onset at between 4 and 6 years. Other papers describing single cases in childhood were published by Levin (1890), Friedmann (1892), Mannheimer (1899), and Zimmer (1899). Cases with an onset during puberty have been described by Kirn (1878; age of onset 14 years, 16 years), von Krafft-Ebing (1888; 14 years), Emmingshaus (1887; 14, 15, 17 years), Pilcz (1901; 12 years). A most comprehensive textbook was written by Emmingshaus (1887), and a later review of the literature was given by Lackmann (1906).

The literature of this century was reviewed by McHarg (1954) and by Hassanyeh and Davison (1980). Kraepelin (1921) estimated a rate of 0.4% for mania with an onset before age 10. Most of the cases in the literature cover the age group 10–19, e.g., single cases aged 11 (Dussik 1934; McHarg 1954), 12 years (Anthony and Scott 1960), 14 years (Rice 1944), and 15 years (White and O'Shanick 1977; Berg et al. 1974). Several cases, again with an age of onset at between 10 and 19, were described by Kasanin and Kaufman (1929), Kasanin (1931), Carter (1942), Campbell (1952), Hudgens (1974), Weinberg and Brumback (1976), Weizman et al. (1979), and Hassanyeh and Davison (1980) with ten cases with an age of onset at 12–15 years. Other adolescent cases were described by Landolt (1957), Annesley (1961), Olsen (1961), and King and Pittman (1969). Campbell (1952) described 18 patients (6 bipolars, 10 unipolar depressives), whose age of onset varied between 6 and 16 years. Olsen (1961) reported 28 cases, de la Cruz (1972) 24 cases, and Boeters (1980) 68 cases. It is obvious that the more recent reports comprise larger samples, and that the affective disorders are no longer considered to be rare among adolescents.

The diagnosis is often difficult (Hassanyeh and Davison 1980), even if the symptoms are more or less the same (Stransky 1911). The first diagnosis is frequently schizophrenia (Carlson and Strober 1978a, b, 1979; Boeters 1980; Joyce 1984; Kendell 1985), or hysteria and encephalitis (Olsen 1961), adjustment reaction (Carlson and Strober 1979), or hyperactivity in children (White and O'Shanick 1977). One case was described as having started with anorexia (Berg et al. 1974). Especially the first episode of mania is frequently misdiagnosed as schizophrenia or hebephrenia (Zeh 1956). A high incidence of schizophreniform symptoms among manic adolescents has been mentioned by Ballenger et al. (1982).

About one-third of major affective disorders seem to begin with cyclothymia (Akiskal et al. 1977) or, in general, with minor affective disorder (Friedman et al. 1983). There is good agreement that adolescents have the same symptoms as adults (Emmingshaus 1887; Ziehen 1917; Friedmann 1909; Coryell and Norten 1980). King and Pittman (1969) followed 21 cases of affective disorders in adolescence over 6 years. The diagnostic stability was high.

The premorbid personality may be cyclothymic and difficult to distinguish from the onset of the illness (Campbell 1952). Patients were also described as being insecure, anxious, and sensitive in childhood (Huhn and Pauly 1973), or in general deviant, queer, stubborn, obstinate, and difficult to get on with (Olsen 1961), or staying home, being insecure, infantile, and irritable (Boeters 1980). Hudgens (1974) found no typical picture in the premorbid personality of 13 bipolar adolescents, while the 25 unipolars he studied were frequently moody, easily discouraged, obsessional, and suffering from recurrent suicidal thoughts. De la Cruz (1972) described an irritable, obstinate, and careless behavior.

According to Carlson et al. (1977), the earliest episode is often atypical and therefore difficult to diagnose. They could not distinguish their adolescents with an onset earlier than 20 from late-onset cases ($n=45$) in terms of sex ratio, number of episodes per year, and outcome. This is at variance with some work by Taylor and Abrams (1973) who tried to distinguish between early and late onset affective disorders. But it is in agreement with Winokur's study of adolescents and late-onset patients over 30 (Winokur 1975).

Outcome is similar to that of adults (Campbell 1952), but an early onset is linked with a double handicap during adolescence interfering with intellectual and personality development which may have repercussions throughout adult life (Hassanyeh and Davison 1980). One-fourth (Carlson et al. 1977) to 36% (Olsen 1961) may become disabled. Sometimes the psychosis starts with a stormy 1 or 2 years and improves considerably again (Hassanyeh and Davison 1980; Boeters (1980). However, Boeters found in 50% of his 68 bipolar cases a malignant course. The earlier the onset, the more recurrent the course – which had already been described by Rehm (1919) and Mauz (1930). Campbell (1952) stressed that in most of the children no precipitation was found. A high relapse rate is characteristic of bipolar psychosis starting in adolsecence (90%), according to Landolt (1957) and Boeters (1980), whereas unipolar mania may have a better prognosis and seems to be more frequent among males (Boeters 1980).

Major depressive disorder frequently starts before age 20 (Puig-Antich and Gittelmann 1982), and its frequency has been estimated at 5% ($n=2694$) by Huhn and Pauly (1973). The first attack can be manic, e.g., in 43% (Olsen 1961), or depressive (Huhn and Pauly 1973). Olsen (1961) found manic attacks to be four times as common as depressive ones until age 18, with a peak at age 17 and a decrease thereafter.

Follow-up studies showed an unfavorable prognosis in four of six cases, as reported by Chess et al. (1983), and a "stable depressive style" in five of ten cases followed over $6^1/_2$ years by Poznanski et al. (1976). Horowitz (1977) described eight cases aged 15–18 with full remission under lithium treatment. He found evidence for precipitating events, and all cases had primarily been diagnosed as schizophrenics. Landolt (1957) followed 60 bipolar patients aged 15–22 over 15–25 years and found no recurrence in 10%; nine patients became catatonic schizophrenic, ten recovered completely, and six had no recurrence following initial hospitalization, whereas all others suffered from recurrent affective disorders. There was not a single suicide.

A recent large study has been published by Kovacs et al. (1984a, b) based on 8- to 13-year-old children who were diagnosed by DSM-III criteria and studied prospectively over 5 years (psychiatric outpatients, patients of an ambulatory medical clinic). The authors compare major affective disorders (MDD), dysthymic disorder (DD), adjustment disorder with depressed mood (ADDM), and nondepressed psychiatric controls. The DD and ADDM groups had an earlier onset than MDD. The mean length of episode of MDD was about 32 weeks, whereas that of DD lasted about 3 years. The recovery rate of the major depressive group ($n=65$) was 92% after $1^1/_2$ years from onset. There was no sex difference in age of onset. The earlier the age of onset of MDD, the more lengthy was the recovery. The authors concluded that there was converging evidence that school-aged children do suffer from depressive disorders, and they confirmed again that the symptoms are similar to those in adult cohorts. The follow-up gave evidence for the assumption that dysthymic disorder and major depressive disorder might be variants of one illness. The course of dysthymia was frequently superimposed by attacks of major depression. The authors concluded that children with dysthymia and/or major depression were at a high risk for a further episode of depressive illness. This conclusion was based on life-table analyses. They also stressed the poor premorbid adjustment of their sample. On the whole, the hypothesis was raised that dysthymic disorder is an early manifestation of affective disorder in preadolescence.

Conclusion

Affective disorders in childhood and adolescence have been extensively described for about two centuries. More recently, there is increasing evidence that both depression and bipolar illness frequently start in the second decade of life. It is often misdiagnosed. There is some evidence that minor affective disorder may later develop into major affective disorder. The rates of recovery and chronicity seem to be comparable to those observed in adults. The social consequences may be more severe, hitting persons early in life. More studies on the premorbid personality and social adjustment would be most desirable in this area. Long-term prospective studies are highly needed.

Needed Areas for Research

Although the course of affective disorders has been the subject of numerous investigations, many questions are still unsolved.

The undifferentiated concept of manic-depressive disorders introduced by Kraepelin (1889) was to a certain extent a step backwards for research in this area, leading to neglect of the distinction between subgroups for decades. Starting from a wide range of affective disorders, future studies should carefully distinguish subgroups, e.g., unipolar and bipolar affective illness, but also subclasses of unipolar depression, e.g., single-episode and recurrent cases, psychotic vs nonpsychotic cases, cases with mood congruent vs mood incongruent psychotic features, primary vs secondary depression, etc. Among bipolar disorders, a distinction should be made not only between bipolar I and bipolar II, but also between single-episode mania and recurrent unipolar mania, bipolar illness dominated by mania, a nuclear group consisting of severe mania and depression, and finally, a preponderantly depressed bipolar group. We do not know much about the prevalence of such subgroups in the normal population. Figures on the ratio between unipolar and bipolar illness should be interpreted critically if they are not based on long observation periods.

In face of the early onset of certain subgroups of affective disorders, the hypothesis has to be tested further whether the illness may actually start as minor affective disorder, hypomania, cyclothymia, dysthymia, minor depression, recurrent brief depression, reactive depression, etc., and later develop into major affective disorder. Future studies should start with representative samples of the normal population at least as from late childhood or adolescence, assessing premorbid personality and social adjustment prior to the onset of illness, and investigating the predictive value of these variables. Much more research is required in the development of instruments to assess specific traits of premorbid personality and minor symptoms of depression and mania. An operational definition of hypomania which is validated by a long follow-up and by genetic findings is needed.

Our knowledge on age of onset is mainly based on retrospective data dependent on the memory of the informants. The first minor manifestations may frequently be overlooked. Age of onset may be an important indicator of heterogeneity of affective disorders. Because most of the studies do not take into account patient samples with a wide age distribution, they usually yield nice one-peak distributions, whereas larger samples including representative samples may show bi- or multimodal distributions. In the future, the presentation of results should give the real distribution, and not unrepresentative means and standard deviations.

Subgroups of affective disorders differ in sex ratio. The interesting facts that females may suffer more frequently from depression and that within the bipolar group the males suffer more from manic syndromes than the females, is of great relevance to biological research. The hypothesis that males may be better protected from becoming depressed than females is highly interesting. Sex differences need more attention in general. They may partly be explained by environmental and biological factors.

The distinction between unipolar depression and bipolar manic-depressive disorder is essential. Their course differs in some variables, e.g., in age of onset, number of episodes, and length of episodes, while it does perhaps not differ in others, e.g., in rates of recovery, chronicity, suicide, percent of lifetime spent in illness, an mortality. Whether the scarcity of differences is real or just an artifact is an open question. Much more prospective research is needed, for instance, in the assessment of minor residual symptoms between episodes. Most of the prospective studies carried out up to now cover only a few years of the course which are in no way representative of the long-term outcome. Few studies exist that assess the social consequences of affective disorders to some extent, and more research in this area must be done. We need more detailed figures about the social career of the patients, the time spent in illness or in treatment over decades. Long-term observations giving percent rates of remission or chronicity frequently neglect deaths due to suicide, or comorbidity with physical illness. We should know more about the preventive effect of maintenance medication not only on future episodes or severity of symptoms, but also on suicide and mortality rates in general.

More research is needed in the field of prediction, but the chief issue is not the search for exotic predictors. Future course is best predicted by past course. More knowledge about the value of a previous history may be obtained from prospective studies. The previous history of the illness is a prerequisite to the selection of the right patient for the right treatment. At the other end of a long-term medication is still the question of when it can safely be discontinued; in face of the possible "burning out" of a group with unipolar depression, this question is of high practical value. Furthermore, we need extensive information about the recurrence of early- and late-onset affective illness in elderly patients in answer to the question of how long they should be maintained on prophylactic medication.

Most of the samples studied up to now were recruited from psychiatric institutions and include mainly inpatients. Fewer studies are based on outpatients, and not much is known about the course of patients with affective disorders treated in general practice over decades. Longitudinal population surveys with repeated measurements would be most important. Such studies require much time, money, and staff, but may turn out to be far more relevant and representative than any other work in this field. They could give not only important information about the course of treated and untreated cases, but also on the influence of personality, environmental factors, and, if assessed, biological variables.

References

Achté KA (1973) Depression und Suizid. Einige prognostische Untersuchungen. Therapiewoche 23:4368–4379

Akiskal HS (1982) Factors associated with incomplete recovery in primary depressive illness. J Clin Psychiatry 43:266–271

Akiskal HS, Djenderedjian AH, Rosenthal RH, Khani MK (1977) Cyclothymic disorder: validating criteria for inclusion in the bipolar affective group. Am J Psychiatry 134:1227–1233

Akiskal HS, Bitar AH, Puzantian VR, Rosenthal TL, Walker PW (1978) The nosological status of neurotic depression. A prospective three- to four-year follow-up examination in light of the primary-secondary and unipolar-bipolar dichotomies. Arch Gen Psychiatry 35:756–766

Akiskal HS, Walker P, Puzantian VR, King D, Rosenthal TL, Dranon M (1983) Bipolar outcome in the course of depressive illness. Phenomenologic, familial, and pharmacologic predictors. J Affective Disord 5:115–128

Angst J (1966) Zur Aetiologie und Nosologie endogener depressiver Psychosen. Eine genetische, soziologische und klinische Studie. Springer, Berlin Heidelberg New York (Monographien aus dem Gesamtgebiete der Neurologie und Psychiatrie, Heft 112)

Angst J (1978) The course of affective disorders. II. Typology of bipolar manic-depressive illness. Arch Psychiatr Nervenkr 226:65–73

Angst J (1980a) Verlauf unipolar depressiver, bipolar manisch-depressiver und schizo-affektiver Erkrankungen und Psychosen. Ergebnisse einer prospektiven Studie. Fortschr Neurol Psychiatr 48:3–30

Angst J (1980b) Clinical typology of bipolar illness. In: Belmaker RH, van Praag HM (eds) Mania – an evolving concept. Spectrum, Jamaica New York, pp 61–76

Angst J (1981) Clinical indications for a prophylactic treatment of depression. In: Mendlewicz J, Coppen A, van Praag HM (eds) Depressive illness – biological and psychopharmacological issues. Symposium Amsterdam 1980 (Advances in biological psychiatry, vol 7). Karger, Basel, pp 218–229

Angst J (1984) A prospective study on the course of affective disorders. In: Mood disorders. Pharmacologic prevention of recurrences. Consensus Development Conference. National Institute of Mental Health, Washington, DC, pp 23–26

Angst J (1985a) Verlauf und Ausgang affektiver und schizo-affektiver Erkrankungen. 2. Weitbrecht-Symposium, Bonn

Angst J (1985b) Switch from depression to mania – a record study over decades between 1920 and 1982. Psychopathology 18:140–154

Angst J, Frey R (1976) Die Prognose endogener Depressionen jenseits des 40. Lebensjahres. Zentralbl Ges Neurol Psychiatr 215:235

Angst J, Weis P (1967) Periodicity of depressive psychoses. In: Brill H, Cole JO, Deniker P, Hippius H, Bradley PB (eds) Neuro-psychopharmacology. Proceedings of the Fifth International Congress of the Collegium Internationale Neuro-Psychopharmacologicum, Washington, DC, 1966. Excerpta Medica, Amsterdam New York, pp 703–710 (International Congress Series, No. 129)

Angst J, Grof P, Hippius H, Poeldinger W, Weis P (1968) La psychose maniaco-dépressive est-elle périodique ou intermittente? Dans: de Ajuriaguerra J (ed) Cycles biologiques et psychiatrie. Symposium Bel-Air III, Genève 1967. Georg, Genève, Masson, Paris, pp 339–351

Angst J, Baastrup PC, Grof P, Hippius H, Pöldinger W, Varga E, Weis P, Wyss F (1973a) Statistische Aspekte des Beginns und Verlaufs schizophrener Psychosen. In: Huber G (ed) Verlauf und Ausgang schizophrener Erkrankungen. 2. Weissenauer Schizophrenie-Symposion. Schattauer, Stuttgart New York, pp 67–78

Angst J, Baastrup PC, Grof P, Hippius H, Pöldinger W, Weis P (1973b) The course of monopolar depression and bipolar psychoses. Psychiatr Neurol Neurochir 76:489–500

Angst J, Felder W, Frey R, Stassen HH (1978) The course of affective disorders. I. Change of diagnosis of monopolar, unipolar, and bipolar illness. Arch Psychiatr Nervenkr 226:57–64

Angst J, Dobler-Mikola A, Hagnell O (1985) How many, and which patients with affective disorders need long-term maintenance therapy? In: Costa E et al. (eds) Chronic treatments in neuropsychiatry. Raven Press, New York, pp 169–172

Annesley PT (1961) Psychiatric illness in adolescence: presentation and prognosis. J Ment Sci 107:268–278

Anthony J, Scott P (1960) Manic-depressive psychosis in childhood. J Child Psychol Psychiatry 1:52–72

Astrup C, Fossum A, Holmboe R (1959) A follow-up study of 270 patients with acute affective psychoses. Acta Psychiatr Scand [Suppl 135]:1–65
Avery D, Winokur G (1976) Mortality in depressed patients treated with electroconvulsive therapy and antidepressants. Arch Gen Psychiatry 33:1029–1037
Baastrup PC, Poulsen JC, Schou M, Thomsen K, Amdisen A (1970) Prophylactic lithium: double-blind discontinuation in manic-depressive and recurrent-depressive disorders. Lancet II:326–330
Baldwin JA (1980) Schizophrenia and physical disease: a preliminary analysis of the data from the Oxford Record Linkage Study. In: Hemmings G (ed) Biochemistry of schizophrenia and addiction. In search of a common factor. MTP Press, Lancaster, pp 297–318
Ballenger JC, Reus VI, Post RM (1982) The "atypical" clinical picture of adolescent mania. Am J Psychiatry 139:602–606
Baron M, Risch N, Mendlewicz J (1983) Age at onset in bipolar-related major affective illness: clinical and genetic implications. J Psychiatr Res 17:5–18
Barthomeuf (1888) Considérations sur les folies intermittentes. Thèse Médicale, Paris
Berg I, Hullin R, Alropp M, O'Brien P, MacDonald R (1974) Bipolar manic depressive psychosis in early adolescence: a case report. Br J Psychiatry 125:416–417
Berger H (1909) Klinische Beiträge zur Melancholie-Frage. Monatsschr Psychiatr Neurol 26:95–112
Berkhan (1863) Irresein bei Kindern. Correspondenzbl Dtsch Gesellsch Psychiatr 10:65–76
Berti Ceroni G, Neri C, Pezzoli A (1984) Chronicity in major depression. A naturalistic prospective study. J Affective Disord 7:123–132
Bland RC, Orn H (1982) Course and outcome in affective disorders. Can J Psychiatry 27:573–578
Boeters U (1980) Zum Verlauf jugendlicher Manien. In: Schimmelpenning GW (ed) Psychiatrische Verlaufsforschung. Methoden und Ergebnisse. Huber, Bern Stuttgart Wien, pp 195–207
Bond ED, Braceland FJ (1937) Prognosis in mental disease. The use of one-page abstracts. Am J Psychiatry 94:263–274
Bornstein PE, Clayton PJ, Halikas JA et al. (1973) The depression of widowhood after thirteen months. Br J Psychiatry 122:561–566
Boyd JH, Weissman MM (1981) Epidemiology of affective disorders. A reexamination and future directions. Arch Gen Psychiatry 38:1039–1046
Bratfos O, Haug JO (1968) Course of manic-depressive psychosis. A follow-up investigation of 215 patients. Acta Psychiatr Scand 44:89–112
Breitenmoser R (1971) Zum Verlauf depressiver Psychosen. Med Diss, Zürich
Brockington IF, Helzer JE, Hillier VF, Francis AF (1982) Definitions of depression: concordance and prediction of outcome. Am J Psychiatry 139:1022–1027
Brown GW, Harris T (1978) Social origins of depression. A study of psychiatric disorder in women. Tavistock, London
Buerger-Prinz H (1961) Probleme der phasischen Psychosen. Enke, Stuttgart (Forum der Psychiatrie, No. 2)
Bunney WE Jr, Murphy DL, Goodwin FK, Borge GF (1972) The "switch process" in manic-depressive illness. I. A systematic study of sequential behavioral changes. Arch Gen Psychiatry 27:295–302
Campbell JD (1952) Manic depressive psychosis in children. Report of 18 cases. J Nerv Ment Dis 116:424–439
Carlson GA, Strober M (1978 a) Affective disorder in adolescence: issues in misdiagnosis. J Clin Psychiatry 39:59, 63–66
Carlson GA, Strober M (1978 b) Manic-depressive illness in early adolescence. A study of clinical and diagnostic characteristics in six cases. J Am Acad Child Psychiatry 17:138–153
Carlson GA, Strober M (1979) Affective disorders in adolescence. Psychiatr Clin North Am 2:511–526

Carlson GA, Kotin J, Davenport JB, Adland M (1974) Follow-up of 53 bipolar manic-depressive patients. Br J Psychiatry 124:134–139
Carlson GA, Davenport YB, Jamison K (1977) A comparison of outcome in adolescent and late onset bipolar manic depressive illness. Am J Psychiatry 134:919–922
Carter AB (1942) The prognostic factor of adolescent psychoses. J Ment Sci 88:31–81
Cassano GB, Maggini C, Akiskal HS (1983) Short-term, subchronic, and chronic sequelae of affective disorders. Psychiatr Clin North Am 6:55–67
Chess S, Thomas A, Hassibi M (1983) Depression in childhood and adolescence. A prospective study of six cases. J Nerv Ment Dis 171:411–420
Ciompi L (1973) Allgemeine Depressionsprobleme im Lichte von Verlaufsforschungen bis ins Alter. Z Gerontol 6:400–408
Ciompi L, Medvecka J (1976) Etude comparative de la mortalité à long terme dans les maladies mentales. Schweiz Arch Neurol Neurochir Psychiatr 118:111–135
Clancy J, Tsuang MT, Norton B, Winokur G (1974) The Iowa 500: a comprehensive study of mania, depression and schizophrenia. J Iowa Med Soc 64:394–398
Clayton PJ (1978) Bipolar affective disorder – techniques and results of treatment. Am J Psychother 32:81–92
Clayton PJ (1980) Discussion of Klerman's paper. (Klerman GJ: Long-term outcome of neurotic depressions) In: Sells SB, Crandall R, Roff M, Strauss JS, Pollin W (eds) Human functioning in longitudinal perspective. Studies of normal and psychopathic populations. Williams and Wilkins, Baltimore London, pp 70–73
Clayton PJ (1981) The epidemiology of bipolar affective disorder. Compr Psychiatry 22:31–43
Clayton PJ (1983a) The prevalence and course of the affective disorders. In: Davis JM, Maas JW (eds) The affective disorders. American Psychiatric Press, Washington, DC, pp 193–201
Clayton PJ (1983b) Epidemiologic and risk factors in suicide. In: Grinspoon L (ed) Psychiatry update, vol II. American Psychiatric Press, Washington, DC, pp 428–434
Clayton PJ (1984) Overview of recurrent mood disorders: definitions and natural course. In: Mood disorders. Pharmacologic prevention of recurrences. Consensus Development Conference, National Institute of Mental Health, Washington, DC, pp 16–22
Clayton PJ, Pitts FN Jr, Winokur G (1965) Affective disorder. IV. Mania. Compr Psychiatry 6:313–322
Cole M, Hicking T (1976) Frequency and significance of minor organic signs in elderly depressives. Can Psychiatr Ass J 21:7–12
Conrad K (1958) Die beginnende Schizophrenie. Versuch einer Gestaltanalyse des Wahns. Thieme, Stuttgart
Coryell W, Norten S (1980) Mania during adolescence. The pathoplastic significance of age. J Nerv Ment Dis 168:611–613
Coryell W, Winokur G (1980) Diagnosis, family, and follow-up studies. In: Belmaker HJ, van Praag HM (eds) Mania – an evolving concept. Spectrum, Jamaica New York, pp 25–41
Coryell W, Winokur G (1982) Course and outcome. In: Paykel ES (ed) Handbook of affective disorders. Churchill Livingstone, Edinburgh London Melbourne New York, pp 93–106
Coryell W, Noyes R, Clancy J (1983) Panic disorder and primary unipolar depression. J Affective Disord 5:311–317
Court JH (1968) Manic-depressive psychosis: an alternative conceptual model. Br J Psychiatry 114:1523–1530
Crowe RR, Smouse PE (1977) The genetic implications of age-dependent penetrance in manic-depressive illness. J Psychiatr Res 13:273–285
de la Cruz N (1972) Manisch-depressives Kranksein bei Jugendlichen zwischen 16 und 19 Jahren. Schweiz Arch Neurol Neurochir Psychiatr 110:279–316
Cutler NR, Post RM (1982) Life course of illness in untreated manic-depressive patients. Compr Psychiatry 23:101–115
D'Elia G, Perris C (1969) Selbstmordversuche im Laufe unipolarer und bipolarer Depressionen. Arch Psychiatr Nervenkr 212:339–356

Derby IM (1933) Manic-depressive "exhaustion" deaths. Psychiatr Q 7:435–449
Dunn G, Skuse D (1981) The natural history of depression in general practice: stochastic models. Psychol Med 11:755–764
Dunner DL, Fleiss JL, Fieve RR (1976) The course of development of mania in patients with recurrent depression. Am J Psychiatry 133:905–908
Dussik KT (1934) Manisch-depressive Psychose bei einem elfjährigen Kind. Psychiatr Neurol Wochenschr 36:305–308
Egeland JA, Hostetter AM (1983) Amish Study I: Affective disorders among the Amish 1976–1980. Am J Psychiatry 140:56–61
Emmingshaus H (1887) Die psychischen Störungen des Kindesalters. Verlag der Laupp'schen Buchhandlung, Tübingen
Endicott J, Andreasen N, Clayton PJ (1980) Bipolar II: combine or keep separate. Sci Proc of APA Convention, San Francisco
van Erp Taalmann Kip MJ (1898) Akute Manie. Allg Z Psychiatr 54:119–135
Evans NJR, Whitlock FA (1983) Mortality and late-onset affective disorder. J Affective Disord 5:297–304
Evans NJR, Baldwin JA, Gath D (1974) The incidence of cancer among inpatients with affective disorders. Br J Psychiatry 124:518–525
Falret JP (1851) De la folie circulaire ou forme de maladie mentale caracterisée par l'alternative régulière de la manie et de la mélancolie. Bull Acad Med (Paris)
Fleiss JL, Dunner DL, Stallone F, Fieve RR (1976) The life table: a method for analyzing longitudinal studies. Arch Gen Psychiatry 33:107–112
Fleiss JL, Prien RF, Dunner DL, Fieve RR (1978) Actuarial studies of the course of manic-depressive illness. Compr Psychiatry 19:355–362
Forssman H, Jansson B (1960) Follow-up study of 849 men admitted for mental disorders to the psychiatric ward of a general hospital. Acta Psychiatr Scand 35:57–72
Fowler RC, Tsuang MT, Kronfol Z (1979) Communication of suicidal intent and suicide in unipolar depression. A forty-year follow-up. J Affective Disord 1:219–225
Frangos E, Athanassenas G, Tsitdourides S, Psilolignos P, Robos A, Katsanou N, Bulgaris C (1980) Seasonality of the episodes of recurrent affective psychoses: possible prophylactic interventions. J Affective Disord 2:239–247
Friedman RC, Hurt SW, Clarkin FJ, Corn R (1983) Primary and secondary affective disorders in adolescents and young adoults. Acta Psychiatr Scand 67:226–235
Friedmann M (1892) Über Nervosität und Psychosen im Kindesalter. MMW 39:359–361, 388–392
Friedmann M (1909) Zur Kenntnis der affektiven Psychosen des Kindesalters, insbesondere der milderen Formen. Monatsschr Psychiatr Neurol 26:36–52
Fukuda K, Etoh T, Iwadate T, Ishii A (1983) The course and prognosis of manic-depressive psychosis: a quantitative analysis of episodes and intervals. Tohoku J Exp Med 139:299–307
Fuller RG (1935) What happens to mental patients after discharge from hospital. Psychiatr Q 9:95–104
Gangil OP, Kumar A, Yadav BS, Jain RK (1982) Family history of mental illness as a factor in relapse and non relapse of discharged functional psychotics. Indian J Psychiatry 24:84–87
Glassner B, Haldipur CV, Dessauersmith J (1979) Role loss and working-class manic depression. J Nerv Ment Dis 167:530–541
Glatzel J, Lungershausen E (1970) Phasenüberdauernde Befindlichkeitsstörungen bei cyclothymen Depressionen. Arch Psychiatr Nervenkr 213:388–395
Goodwin FK, Jamison KR (1984) The natural course of manic-depressive illness. In: Post RM, Ballenger JC (eds) The neurobiology of the mood disorders. Williams and Wilkins, Baltimore
Griesinger W (1845) Pathologie und Therapie der psychischen Krankheiten für Ärzte und Studierende, 1st edn. Krabbe, Stuttgart

Grof P, Angst J, Haines T (1974) The clinical course of depression: practical issues. In: Angst J (ed) Classification and prediction of outcome of depression. Symposium, Schloss Reinhartshausen/Rhein 1973. Schattauer, Stuttgart New York, pp 141–148 (Symposia Medica Hoechst, No. 8)
Guze SB, Robins E (1970) Suicide and primary affective disorder. Br J Psychiatry 117:437–438
Hagnell O, Lanke J, Rosman B (1981) Suicide rates in the Lundby study: mental illness as a risk factor for suicide. Neuropsychobiology 7:248–253
Hassanyeh F, Davison K (1980) Bipolar affective psychosis with onset before age 16 years. Report of 10 cases. Br J Psychiatry 137:530–539
Hastings DW (1958) Follow-up results in psychiatric illness. Am J Psychiatry 114:1057–1066
Heimbuch RC, Matthysse S, Kidd KK (1980) Estimating age-of-onset distributions for disorders with variable onset. Am J Hum Genet 32:564–574
Hinrichsen O (1898) Statistischer Beitrag zur Frage nach der Häufigkeit der einfachen akuten Manie im Verhältnis zu den periodischen Formen derselben. Allg Z Psychiatr 54:786–805
Hopkinson G (1963) The onset of affective illness. Psychiatr Neurol (Basel) 146:133–140
Hopkinson G, Ley P (1969) A genetic study of affective disorder. Br J Psychiatry 115:917–922
Hornstra RK, Klassen D (1977) The course of depression. Compr Psychiatry 18:119–125
Horowitz HA (1977) Lithium and the treatment of adolescent manic-depressive illness. Dis Nerv Syst 38:480–483
von Hösslin C (1909) Beitrag zur Kenntnis des Verlaufes und Ausganges des manisch-depressiven Irreseins. Zentralbl Nervenheilk Psychiatr 32:823–829
Huba GJ, Lawlor WG, Stallone F, Fieve RR (1976) The use of autocorrelation analysis in the longitudinal study of mood patterns in depressed patients. Br J Psychiatry 128:146–155
Huber G (1966) Reine Defektsyndrome und Basisstadien endogener Psychosen. Fortschr Neurol Psychiatr 34:409–426
Hudgens RW (1974) Psychiatric disorders in adolescents. Williams and Wilkins, Baltimore
Huhn A, Pauly U (1973) Klinik, Verlauf und Prognose der Zyklothymie bei Jugendlichen. In: Kranz H, Heinrich K (eds) Chronische endogene Psychosen. 6. Bad Kreuznacher Symposium 1972. Thieme, Stuttgart, pp 17–31
Huston PE, Locher LM (1948 a) Involutional psychosis. Course when untreated and when treated with electric shock. Arch Neurol Psychiatry 59:385–394
Huston PE, Locher LM (1948 b) Manic-depressive psychosis. Course when treated and untreated with electric shock. Arch Neurol Psychiatry 60:37–48
Jacoby RJ (1981) Depression in the elderly. Br J Hosp Med (January):40–47
Janzarik W (1959) Dynamische Grundkonstellationen in endogenen Psychosen. Ein Beitrag zur Differentialtypologie der Wahnphänomene. Springer, Berlin Göttingen Heidelberg (Monographien aus dem Gesamtgebiete der Neurologie und Psychiatrie, Heft 86)
Johnson GFS, Hunt GE (1979) Onset of mania in bipolar manic-depressive patients. Aust NZ J Psychiatry 13:57–61
Johnson GFS, Leeman MM (1977) Onset of illness in bipolar manic-depressives and their affectively ill first-degree relatives. Biol Psychiatry 12:733–741
Jones BD, Steinberg S, Chouinard G (1984) Fast-cycling bipolar disorder induced by withdrawal from long-term treatment with a tricyclic antidepressant. Am J Psychiatry 141:108–109
Joyce PR (1984) Age of onset in bipolar affective disorder and misdiagnosis as schizophrenia. Psychol Med 14:145–149
Kasanin J (1931) The affective psychoses in children. Am J Psychiatry 10:897–926
Kasanin J, Kaufman MR (1929) A study of the functional psychoses in childhood. Am J Psychiatry 9:307-384

Kawashima K (1979) Clinical studies of depressive illness in old age. (Japanese with Engl. summary) Tokyo Jikeikai Med J 94:365–376

Kay DWK (1962) Outcome and cause of death in mental disorders of old age: a long-term follow-up of functional and organic psychoses. Acta Psychiatr Scand 38:249–276

Kay DWK, Bergmann K (1966) Physical disability and mental health in old age. A follow-up of a random sample of elderly people seen at home. J Psychosom Res 10:3–12

Kay DWK, Garside RF, Roy JR, Beamish P (1969) "Endogenous" and "neurotic" syndromes of depression: a 5- to 7-year follow-up of 104 cases. Br J Psychiatry 155:389–399

Keller MB, Shapiro RW (1981) Major depressive disorder. Initial results from a one-year prospective naturalistic follow-up study. J Nerv Ment Dis 169:761–768

Keller MB, Shapiro RW (1982) "Double depression": superimposition of acute depressive episodes on chronic depressive disorders. Am J Psychiatry 139:438–442

Keller MB, Shapiro RW, Lavori PW, Wolfe N (1982a) Relapse in major depressive disorder. Analysis with the life table. Arch Gen Psychiatry 39:911–915

Keller MB, Shapiro RW, Lavori PW, Wolfe N (1982b) Recovery in major depressive disorder. Analysis with the life table and regression models. Arch Gen Psychiatry 39:905–910

Keller MB, Lavori PW, Lewis CE, Klerman GL (1983) Predictors of relapse in major depressive disorder. JAMA 250:3299–3304

Kendell RE (1985) The diagnosis of mania. J Affective Disord 8:207–213

Kerr TA, Schapira K, Roth M (1969) The relationship between premature death and affective disorders. Br J Psychiatry 115:1277–1282

Kerr TA, Roth M, Schapira K, Gurney C (1972) The assessment and prediction of outcome in affective disorders. Br J Psychiatry 121:167–174

Kielholz P (1959) Klinik, Differentialdiagnostik und Therapie der depressiven Zustandsbilder. Documenta Geigy, Basel (Acta Psychosomatica No. 2)

Kimura S, Ohya D, Koh T, Iwamura H (1984) Course and prognosis of endogenous-phasic psychoses in adolescence. Psychopathology 17:137–143

King LJ, Pittman GD (1969) A six-year follow-up study of sixty-five adolescent patients: predictive value of presenting clinical picture. Br J Psychiatry 115:1437–1441

Kinkelin M (1954) Verlauf und Prognose des manisch-depressiven Irreseins. Schweiz Arch Neurol Neurochir Psychiatr 73:100–146

Kirn L (1878) Die periodischen Psychosen; eine klinische Abhandlung. Enke, Stuttgart

Klerman GL (1980) Long-term outcome of neurotic depressions. In: Sells SB, Crandall R, Roff M, Strauss JS, Pollin W (eds) Human functioning in longitudinal perspective. Studies of normal and psychopathic populations. Williams and Wilkins, Baltimore London, pp 58–70

Kovacs M, Rush AJ, Beck AT, Hollon SD (1981) Depressed outpatients treated with cognitive therapy or pharmacotherapy, a one-year follow-up. Arch Gen Psychiatry 38:33–39

Kovacs M, Feinberg TL, Crouse-Novak MA, Paulauskas SL, Finkelstein R (1984a) Depressive disorders in childhood. I. A longitudinal prospective study of characteristics and recovery. Arch Gen Psychiatry 41:229–237

Kovacs M, Feinberg TL, Crouse-Novak MA, Paulauskas SL, Pollock M, Finkelstein R (1984b) Depressive disorders in childhood. II. A longitudinal study of the risk for a subsequent major depression. Arch Gen Psychiatry 41:643–649

Kraepelin E (1889) Psychiatrie. Ein lehrbuch für Studierende und Ärzte, 3rd edn. Barth, Leipzig

Kraepelin E (1913) Das manisch-depressive Irresein. In: Psychiatrie. Ein Lehrbuch für Studierende und Ärzte, vol 3, part 2. Barth, Leipzig, pp 1183–1395

Kraepelin E (1921) Manic-depressive insanity. In: Wolpert EA (ed) Manic-depressive illness. History of a syndrome. International Universities Press, New York 1977, pp 33–111

von Krafft-Ebing R (1888) Lehrbuch der Psychiatrie auf klinischer Grundlage für praktische Ärzte und Studierende, 3rd edn. Enke, Stuttgart

Krauthammer C, Klerman GL (1979) The epidemiology of mania. In: Shopsin B (ed) Manic illness. Raven Press, New York, pp 11–28
Kreuser H (1900) Spätgenesungen bei Geisteskrankheiten. Allg Z Psychiatr 57:771–813
Kukopoulos A, Caliari B, Tundo A, Minnai G, Floris G, Reginaldi D, Tondo L (1983) Rapid cyclers, temperament, and antidepressants. Compr Psychiatry 24:249–258
Lackmann W (1906) Über manisch-depressives Irresein im Kindesalter. Med Diss, Erlangen
Lambranzi, Perazzolo (1906) Le recidive nella freniatria manica-depressiva. Giorn Psich Clin Tec Man
Landolt AB (1957) Follow-up studies on circular manic-depressive reactions occurring in the young. Bull NY Acad Med 33:65–73
Langelüddeke A (1941) Über Lebenserwartung und Rückfallhäufigkeit bei Manisch-Depressiven. Z Psych Hygiene 14:1–15
Lauter H (1969) Phasenüberdauernder Persönlichkeitswandel und persistierende Symptome bei der endogenen Depression. In: Hippius H, Selbach H (eds) Das depressive Syndrom. Int. Symposion, Berlin 1968. Urban und Schwarzenberg, München Berlin Wien, pp 128–132
Lavori PW, Keller MB (1983) Application of survival analysis to psychiatric research. In: Gibbons RD, Dysken MW (eds) Statistical and methodological advances in psychiatric research. Spectrum, New York
Lavori PW, Keller MB, Klerman GL (1984) Relapse in affective disorders: a reanalysis of the literature using life table methods. J Psychiatr Res 18:13–25
Leonhard K, Korff I, Schulz H (1962) Die Temperamente in den Familien der monopolaren und bipolaren phasischen Psychosen. Psychiatr Neurol (Basel) 143:416–434
Lerer B, Birmacher B, Ebstein RP, Belmaker RH (1980) 48-hour depressive cycling induced by antidepressant. Br J Psychiatry 137:183–185
Levin (1890) Über periodische Manie. Med Diss, Strassbourg
Lewinsohn PM, Fenn DS, Stanton AK, Franklin J (unpublished) Relationship of age at onset to duration of episode in unipolar depression
Lewis JL, Winokur G (1982) The induction of mania. A natural history study with controls. Arch Gen Psychiatry 39:303–306
Lilliker SL (1980) Prevalence of diabetes in a manic-depressive population. Compr Psychiatry 21:270–275
Lönnqvist J, Koskenvuo M, Kapiro J, Langinvainio H (1983) The mortality in psychiatric disorders: a three-year prospective follow-up study. In: Soubrier JP, Vedrinne J (eds) Dépression et suicide. Aspects médicaux, psychologiques et socio-culturels. C. R. de la XIe réunion de l'association internationale pour la prévention du suicide, Paris 1981. Pergamon Press, Paris Oxford New York Toronto Sidney Frankfurt, pp 198–203
Loranger AW, Levine PM (1978) Age at onset of bipolar affective illness. Arch Gen Psychiatry 35:1345–1348
Luce GG (1973) Body time – the natural rhythms of the body. Paladin, St Albans (cit: Aretaeus, c. 600 BC)
Lundquist G (1945) Prognosis and course in manic-depressive psychoses: a follow-up study of 319 first admissions. Acta Psychiatr Scand [Suppl 35]:1–96
MacDonald JB (1918) Prognosis in manic-depressive insanity. J Nerv Ment Dis 47:20–30
MacVane JR, Lange JD, Brown WA, Zayat M (1978) Psychological functioning of bipolar manic-depressives in remission. Arch Gen Psychiatry 35:1351–1354
Malzberg B (1929) A statistical study of the factor of age in the manic-depressive psychoses. Psychiatr Q 3:590–604
Mannheimer (1899) Les troubles mentaux de l'enfance. Paris
Matussek P, Halbach A, Troeger U (1965) Endogene Depression. Eine statistische Untersuchung unbehandelter Fälle. Urban und Schwarzenberg, München Berlin
Mauz F (1930) Die Prognostik der endogenen Psychosen. Thieme, Leipzig
Mayser (1899) Beitrag zur Lehre von der Manie. (Sitzungsbericht) Arch Psychiatr 31:500–502

McHarg JF (1954) Mania in childhood. Arch Neurol Psychiatry 72:531–539
Mendel E (1881) Die Manie. Urban und Schwarzenberg, Wien Leipzig
Mendlewicz J, Fieve RR, Rainer JD, Fleiss JL (1972) Manic-depressive illness: a comparative study of patients with and without a family history. Br J Psychiatry 120:523–530
Merikangas KR, Bromet EJ, Spiker DG (1983) Assortative mating, social adjustment, and course of illness in primary affective disorder. Arch Gen Psychiatry 40:795–800
Meyer L (1874) Über zirkuläre Geisteskrankheiten. Arch Psychiatr 4:139–158
Milenkov K, Apostolov W (1969) Zur Frage der chronischen Verläufe bei Zyklophrenie. (Bulgarisch) Bull NIINP Sofia 13:81–86
Mirin SM, Schatzberg AF, Creasey DE (1981) Hypomania and mania after withdrawal of tricyclic antidepressants. Am J Psychiatry 138:87–89
Mitchell SW (1897) An analysis of 3000 cases of melancholia. Trans Assoc Am Physicians 12:480–487
Morrison JR, Winokur G, Crowe R, Clancy J (1973) The Iowa 500: The first follow-up. Arch Gen Psychiatry 29:678–682
Murphy E (1983) The prognosis of depression in old age. Br J Psychiatry 142:111–119
Murphy GE, Woodruff RA, Herjanic M (1974a) The validation of specific diagnostic criteria for primary affective disorder by means of a blind five year follow-up. J Psychiatr Res 10:321–322
Murphy GE, Woodruff RA Jr, Herjanic M, Fischer JR (1974b) Validity of the diagnosis of primary affective disorder. A prospective study with a five-year follow-up. Arch Gen Psychiatry 30:751–756
Murphy GE, Woodruff RA Jr, Herjanic M, Super G (1974c) Variability of the clinical course of primary affective disorder. Arch Gen Psychiatry 30:757–761
Myers JK, Weissman MM, Tischler GL, Holzer CE III, Leaf PJ, Orvaschel H, Anthony JC, Boyd JH, Burke JD Jr, Kramer M, Stoltzman R (1984) Six-month prevalence of psychiatric disorders in three communities: 1980–1982. Arch Gen Psychiatry 41:959–967
Nandi DN, Banerjee G, Ganguli H, Ajmany S, Boral GC, Gosh A, Sarkar S (1978) The natural history of mental disorders in a rural community. A longitudinal field-survey. Indian J Psychiatry 21:390–396
Nasr S, Altman EG, Meltzer HY (1981) Concordance of atopic and affective disorders. J Affective Disord 3:291–296
Nitsche P (1910) Über chronisch-manische Zustände. Zugleich ein Beitrag zur Lehre von den krankhaften Persönlichkeiten. Allg Z Psychiatr 67:36–133
Nöthig V, Jerbic B, Baldauf V (1973) Analysis of manic-depressive psychoses treated in the last five years (1968–1972). Abstract 3rd Yugoslav Psychopharmacol Symposium, Opatija, p 176
Nuller YL, Kalinin OM, Rubtsova SK (1972) The use of factor analysis for the study of the course of manic-depressive psychosis. Zh Nevropathol Psikhiatr 72:548–554
Nunn CMH (1979) Mixed affective states and the natural history of manic-depressive psychosis. Br J Psychiatry 134:153–160
Olsen T (1961) Follow-up study of manic-depressive patients whose first attack occured before the age of 19. In: Kristiansen ES (ed) Depression. Acta Psychiatr Scand [Suppl] 162:45–51
Oltman JE, Friedman S (1962) Life cycles in patients with manic-depressive psychosis. Am J Psychiatry 119:174–176
Parker G, Walter S (1982) Seasonal variation in depressive disorders and suicidal deaths in New South Wales. Br J Psychiatry 140:626–632
Paskind HA (1930) Manic-depressive psychosis as seen in private praxis. Sex distribution and age incidence of first attacks. Arch Neurol Psychiatry 23:152–158
Paykel ES, Klerman GL, Prusoff BA (1974) Prognosis of depression and the endogenous-neurotic distinction. Psychol Med 4:57–64
Peley D, Vargha M (1974) Veränderungen im Verlauf manisch-depressiver Psychosen. Psychiatr Neurol Med Psychol (Leipz) 26:395–399

Perris C (1966) A study of bipolar (manic-depressive) and unipolar recurrent depressive psychoses. Acta Psychiatr Scand [Suppl 194]:1–189
Perris C (1968) The course of depressive psychoses. Acta Psychiatr Scand 44:238–248
Perris C (1969) The separation of bipolar (manic-depressive) from unipolar recurrent depressive psychoses. Behav Neuropsychiatry 1:17–24
Peselow ED, Dunner DL, Fieve RR, Deutsch SI, Rubinstein ME (1982) Age of onset of affective illness. Psychiatr Clin (Basel) 15:124–132
Petterson U (1977) Manic-depressive illness. A clinical, social and genetic study. Acta Psychiatr Scand [Suppl 269]
Pilcz A (1901) Die periodischen Geistesstörungen. Eine klinische Studie. G Fischer, Jena
Pollock HM (1931 a) Recurrence of attacks in manic-depressive psychoses. Am J Psychiatry 11:567–574
Pollock HM (1931 b) Recurrence of attacks in manic-depressive psychoses. In: White WA, Davis TK, Frantz AM (eds) Manic-depressive psychosis. Williams and Willkins, Baltimore, pp 668–675
Poort R (1945) Catamnestic investigations on manic-depressive psychoses with special reference to the prognosis. Acta Psychiatr Scand 20:59–74
Post F (1962) The significance of affective symptoms in old age. A follow-up study of one hundred patients. Oxford University Press, London New York Toronto (Maudsley Monographs, No. 10)
Post F (1972) The management and nature of depressive illnesses in late life: a follow-through study. Br J Psychiatry 121:393–404
Poznanski EO, Krahenbuhl V, Zrull JP (1976) Childhood depression. A longitudinal perspective. J Am Acad Child Psychiatry 15:491–501
Prien RF, Klett J, Caffey EM (1974) Lithium prophylaxis in recurrent affective illness. Am J Psychiatry 131:198–203
Puig-Antich J, Gittelman R (1982) Depression in childhood and adolescence. In: Paykel ES (ed) The handbook of affective disorders. Churchill Livingstone, Edinburgh London Melbourne New York, pp 379–392
Rao AV, Nammalvar N (1977) The course and outcome in depressive illness. A follow-up study of 122 cases in Madurai, India. Br J Psychiatry 130:392–396
Refsum HE, Astrup C (1980) Reactive depression: a follow-up. Neuropsychobiology 6:79–90
Rehm O (1907) Verlaufsformen des manisch-depressiven Irreseins. Centralbl Nervenheilk Psychiatr 30:480–481
Rehm O (1919) Das manisch melancholische Irresein. (Manisch-depressives Irresein Kraepelin) Springer, Berlin (Monographien aus dem Gesamtgebiete der Neurologie und Psychiatrie, vol 17)
Rennie TAC (1942) Prognosis in manic-depressive psychoses. Am J Psychiatry 98:801–814
Rice KK (1944) Clinical, technical and occasional notes: Regular forty to fifty day cycle of psychotic behavior in a 14 year old boy. Arch Neurol Psychiatry 51:478–480
Rihmer Z (1980) Season of birth and season of hospital admission in bipolar depressed female patients. Psychiatry Res 3:247–251
Robins E, Guze SB (1972) Classification of affective disorders: the primary-secondary, the endogenous-reactive, and the neurotic-psychotic concepts. In: Williams TA, Katz MM, Shield JA Jr (eds) Recent advances in the psychobiology of the depressive illnesses. Proceedings of a Workshop, Clinical Research Branch, Division of Extramural Research Programs, NIMH, Williamsburg, Virgnia 1969. DHEW Publ. No (HSM) 70–9053. Washington, DC, pp 283–293
Robins LN, Helzer JE, Weissman MM, Orvaschel H, Gruenberg E, Burke JD Jr, Regier DA (1984) Lifetime prevalence of specific psychiatric disorders in three sites. Arch Gen Psychiatry 41:949–958
Rosen LN, Rosenthal NE, van Dusen PH, Dunner DL, Fieve RR (1983) Age at onset and number of psychotic symptoms in bipolar I and schizoaffective disorder. Am J Psychiatry 140:1523–1524

Rosenthal NE, Lewy AJ, Wehr TA, Kern HE, Goodwin FK (1983) Seasonal cycling in a bipolar patient. Psychiatry Res 8:25–31
Rosenthal NE, Sack DA, Gillin JC, Lewy AJ, Goodwin FK, Davenport Y, Mueller PS, Newsome DA, Wehr TA (1984) Seasonal affective disorder. A descritpion of the syndrome and preliminary findings with light therapy. Arch Gen Psychiatry 41:72–80
Roth M, Kay DWK (1956) Affective disorder arising in the senium. II: Physical disability as an aetiological factor. J Ment Sci 102:141–150
Saiz G (1907) Untersuchungen über die Ätiologie der Manie, der periodischen Manie und des zirkulären Irreseins, nebst Besprechung einzelner Krankheitssymptome. Karger, Berlin
Saran BM (1971) The course of recurrent depressive illness in selected patients from a defined population. Int Pharmacopsychiatry 5:119–131
Schapira K, Roth M, Kerr TA, Gurney C (1972) The prognosis of affective disorders: the differentiation of anxiety states from depressive illnesses. Br J Psychiatry 121:175–181
Schipkowensky N, Milenkow K (1970) Zur Epidemiologie, Ätiologie und Prophylaxe der chronischen Zyklophrenie. Int Pharmacopsychiatry 4:117–153
Schulz B (1949) Sterblichkeit endogen Geisteskranker und ihrer Eltern. Z Menschl Vererbungs Konstitutionslehre 29:338–367
Shobe FO, Brion P (1971) Long-term prognosis in manic-depressive illness: a follow-up investigation of ill patients. Arch Gen Psychiatry 24:334–337
Shulman K, Post F (1980) Bipolar affective disorder in old age. Br J Psychiatry 136:26–32
Siris SG, Chertoff HR, Perel JM (1979) Rapid-cycling affective disorder during imipramine treatment: a case report. Am J Psychiatry 136:341–342
Slater E (1938 a) Zur Periodik des manisch-depressiven Irreseins. Z Ges Neurol Psychiatr 162:794–801
Slater E (1938 b) Zur Erbpathologie des manisch-depressiven Irreseins. Die Eltern und Kinder von Manisch-Depressiven. Z Ges Neurol Psychiatr 163:1–47
Smeraldi E, Negri F, Melica AM (1977) A genetic study of affective disorders. Acta Psychiatr Scand 56:382–398
Stallone F, Dunner DL, Ahearn J, Fieve RR (1980) Statistical predictions of suicide in depressives. Compr Psychiatry 21:381–387
Steen RR (1933) Prognosis in manic-depressive psychoses. Psychiatr Q 7:419–429
Steiner J (1873) Compendium der Kinderkrankheiten für Studierende und Ärzte, 2nd edn. Vogel, Leipzig
Stenstedt A (1952) A study in manic-depressive psychosis: clinical, social, and genetic investigations. Acta Psychiatr Scand [Suppl 79]:1–112
Stenstedt A (1959) Involutional melancholia. An etiologic, clinical and social study of endogenous depression in later life, with special reference to genetic factors. Acta Psychiatr Scand [Suppl 127]:5–68
Stransky E (1911) Das manisch-depressive Irresein. Deuticke, Leipzig Wien
Supprian U (1973) Perioden im Ablauf phasischer Psychosen. Therapiewoche 23/46:2–5
Supprian U (1975 a) Ein theoretisches Modell für den Gesamtablauf der manisch-depressiven Psychosen. Fortschr Neurol Psychiatr 43:358–379
Supprian U (1975 b) Über eine strenge Periodizität im Ablauf einer manisch-depressiven Psychose. Nervenarzt 46:440–446
Supprian U (1975 c) Über die chronopathologische Struktur einiger langer Katamnesen bei manisch-depressiver Erkrankung. Fortschr Neurol Psychiatr 43:575–601
Supprian U (1977) Verlaufsstudien an einer phasischen Psychose. Fortschr Neurol Psychiatr 45:596–614
Swift HM (1907) The prognosis of recurrent insanity of the manic-depressive type. Am J Insanity 64:311–326
Taschev T (1965) Statistisches über die Melancholie. Fortschr Neurol Psychiatr 33:25–36
Taschev T, Roglev M (1973) Das Schicksal der Melancholiker im fortgeschrittenen Alter. Arch Psychiatr Nervenkr 217:377–386

Taylor MA, Abrams R (1973) Manic states. A genetic study of early and late onset affective disorders. Arch Gen Psychiatry 28:656–658
Taylor MA, Abrams R (1981) Early- and late-onset bipolar illness. Arch Gen Psychiatry 38:58–61
Till E, Vuckovik S (1970) Über den Einfluß der thymoleptischen Behandlung auf den Verlauf endogener Depressionen. Int Pharmacopsychiatry 4:210–219
Tondo L, Laddomada P, Serra G, Minnai G, Kukopulos A (1981) Rapid cyclers and antidepressants. Int Pharmacopsychiatry 16:119–123
Tsuang MT, Winokur G (1974) Bipolar primary affective disorder. J Oper Psychiatry 6:47–53
Tsuang MT, Woolson RF (1977) Mortality in patients with schizophrenia, mania, depression and surgical conditions: a comparison with general population mortality. Br J Psychiatry 130:162–166
Tsuang MT, Woolson RF (1978) Excess mortality in schizophrenia and affective disorders. Do suicides and accidental deaths solely account for this excess? Arch Gen Psychiatry 35:1181–1185
Tsuang MT, Dempsey GM, Rauscher F (1976) A study of "atypical schizophrenia": comparison with schizophrenia and affective disorder by sex, age of admission, precipitant, outcome, and family history. Arch Gen Psychiatry 33:1157–1160
Tsuang MT, Woolson RF, Fleming JA (1979) Long-term outcome of major psychoses. I. Schizophrenia and affective disorders compared with psychiatrically symptom-free surgical conditions. Arch Gen Psychiatry 36:1295–1301
Tsuang MT, Woolson RF, Fleming JA (1980 a) Causes of death in schizophrenia and manic-depression. Br J Psychiatry 136:239–242
Tsuang MT, Woolson RF, Fleming JA (1980 b) Premature deaths in schizophrenia and affective disorders. An analysis of survival curves and variables affecting the shortened survival. Arch Gen Psychiatry 37:979–983
Umenhoff D (1963) Zur Prognose der manisch-depressiven Erkrankungen bei Jugendlichen. Med Diss, Würzburg
Vedrani (1905) Alcuni casi di freniatria manica-depressiva. Giorn di Psich Clin Tecn Man
Walker R (1907) Über manische und depressive Psychosen. Arch Psychiatr Nervenkr 42:788–868
Watts CAH (1956) The incidence and prognosis of endogenous depression. Br Med J I:1392–1397
Wehr TA, Goodwin FK (1979) Rapid cycling in manic-depressives induced by tricyclic antidepressants. Arch Gen Psychiatry 36:555–559
Weinberg WA, Brumback RA (1976) Mania in childhood. Case studies and literature review. Am J Dis Child 130:380–385
Weissman MM, Prusoff BA, Klerman GL (1978) Personality and the prediction of long term outcome of depression. Am J Psychiatry 135:797–800
Weissman MM, Klerman GL, Prusoff BA, Sholomskas D, Padian N (1981) Depressed outpatients. Results one year after treatment with drugs and/or interpersonal psychotherapy. Arch Gen Psychiatry 38:51–55
Weitbrecht HJ (1949) Zyklothymie. Fortschr Neurol Psychiatr 17:437–481
Weitbrecht HJ (1961) Endogene phasische Psychosen. Symptombilder und Verläufe. Fortschr Neurol Psychiatr 29:129–144
Weitbrecht HJ (1967) Die chronische Depression. Wien Z Nervenheilk 24:265–281
Weizman A, Weizman R, Tyano S, Wijsenbeek H (1979) Bipolar depression (manic-depressive disease) in early adolescence. Adolescence 14:617–620
Wertham FI (1929 a) A group of benign chronic psychoses: prolonged manic excitements. With a statistical study of age, duration and frequency in 2000 manic attacks. Am J Psychiatry 9:17–78
Wertham FI (1929 b) Die klinische Kerngruppe der chronischen Manie. Z Gesamte Neurol Psychiatr 121:770–779

White JH, O'Shanick G (1977) Juvenile manic-depressive illness. Am J Psychiatry 134:1035–1036

Winokur G (1970) The natural history of the affective disorders (manias and depression). Semin Psychiatry 2:451–463

Winokur G (1975) The Iowa 500: heterogeneity and course in manic-depressive illness (bipolar). Compr Psychiatry 16:125–131

Winokur G, Clayton PJ (1967) Family history studies. I. Two types of affective disorders separated according to genetic and clinical factors. In: Wortis J (ed) Recent advances in biological psychiatry, vol 9. Plenum Press, New York, pp 35–50

Winokur G, Morrison J (1973) The Iowa 500: follow-up of 225 depressives. Br J Psychiatry 123:543–548

Winokur G, Clayton PJ, Reich T (1969) Manic depressive illness. C. V. Mosby, Saint Louis

Woodruff RA, Guze SB, Clayton PJ (1971) Unipolar and bipolar primary affective disorder. Br J Psychiatry 119:33–38

World Health Organization (1979) Schizophrenia. An international follow-up study. Wiley, Chichester New York Brisbane Toronto

Zeh W (1956) Zur Psychopathologie der zyklothymen Manie. Fortschr Neurol Psychiatr 24:149–160

Zeller E (1844) Bericht über die Wirksamkeit der Heilanstalt Winnenthal vom 1. 3. 1840 bis 28. 2. 1843. Allg Z Psychiatr 1:1–79

Zhenyi X, Mingdao Z, Heqin Y (1980) Affective psychosis. A follow-up, retrospective classification and heredofamilial study. Chin Med J (Peking) 93:365–368

Ziehen T (1896) Die Erkennung und Behandlung der Melancholie in der Praxis. Karl Marhold, Halle

Ziehen T (1917) Die Geisteskrankheiten des Kindesalters einschließlich des Schwachsinns und der psychopathischen Konstitutionen. Reuter and Reichhard, Berlin

Zilborg G (1941) A history of medical psychology. Norton, New York

Zimmer (1899) Ein Fall von infantiler circulärer Psychose. Med Diss, Berlin

Zis AP, Goodwin FK (1979) Major affective disorders as a recurrent illness. Arch Gen Psychiatry 36:835–839

Zis AP, Grof P, Webster M, Goodwin FK (1980) Prediction of relapse in recurrent affective disorder. Psychopharmacol Bull 16:47–49

Ziskind E, Somerfeld-Ziskind E, Ziskind L (1945) Metrazol and electric convulsive therapy of the affective psychoses. A controlled series of observations covering a period of five years. Arch Neurol Psychiatry 53:212–217

Comments

P. Pichot

To discuss Professor Angst's paper is an extremely difficult task. The extent of the literature reviewed, the quality of the analysis, and the caution expressed in the conclusions would be difficult to surpass. In my opinion this paper is probably the best survey of the problem yet written, and, for that reason, I shall not dare to discuss it in the usual sense of the word, but make some remarks on points I consider worthy of further comments.

My first remark will deal with the title, which includes the expression "affective disorders." It is used in the English language, and, as far as I know, under the influence of our American colleagues, to describe the pathological states related to depression and mania. It is however noteworthy that the authors of the now authoritative American nosology, the DSM-III, although adopting "affective disorders," have stressed in a footnote that they are only following a faulty American tradition, and that the correct term would be "mood disorders." I believe that this apparently purely formal problem is of some importance, since it is usually accepted that anxiety states are also, in the true sense of the word, affective disorders, an evident source of confusion. I wonder if it would not be a good initiative to give some help to the authors of the DSM-III, by suggesting that they take the step of substituting mood disorders for affective disorders. If we Europeans adopt the tradition considered as faulty by the Americans themselves, we cannot expect that they will have the courage to reform their nomenclature.

Leaving aside this issue, I am struck in Angst's paper by the magnitude of the methodological problems he has himself discussed with admirable skill, and which in many cases, although the available literature is very extensive, make conclusions extremely difficult to draw. It seems that the two main difficulties are a) the definition of the cases and b) the subgrouping.

Other technical problems are related to the observation technique used (retrospective, follow-up prospective, and concerning selected groups or the whole population), and to the fact that, at the present time, most of the patients receive some sort of treatment. All are evidently interrelated, and in one way or another, are sources of errors in every aspect discussed by Angst.

---

24 Rue des Fossés Saint Jacques, F-75005 Paris

Depressive Illness: Prediction of Course and Outcome
Edited by T. Helgason and R. J. Daly

What is depression, what is mania, and what are their limits with normality and with other pathological states? I do not intend to solve the problem, but in Angst's paper it is obvious that a comparison of the results from different sources is made extremely difficult by the differences in the definitions given – or more often not given. One is confronted with the impossible task to compare cases which have only a small fraction of the total variance in common. The introduction of the diagnostic criteria by the St. Louis School is undoubtedly a great step forward and I personally consider that their adoption by the DSM-III is probably the most important feature of the new American nosological system. I have no intention to discuss here which system of criteria is the best, or how they can be improved, but I believe that one of the urgent tasks is to reach a consensus for future work. The collection of data when one studies the clinical course of the affective disorders is necessarily a tedious task, which can take many years and, if the diagnostic criteria adopted by different studies are not the same, or if they are modified in the course of time – you may be reminded that the DSM-III will appear in a revised form in early 1987, 7 years after the initial publication – we will again be confronted with the same difficulties which are so evident in Angst's paper. If I have made several references to the DSM-III, it is not because I consider the adopted criteria to be good. In fact I consider them as deficient in several respects with regard to affective disorders. But they have introduced a way of thinking and, as I said, one of the urgent tasks is to reach an agreement, even if imperfect.

When it comes to the subdivision of the affective states, we are faced with the same problem, in an even more complex form. In looking at the legend of Table 3 in Angst's paper, it can be seen that the author has managed to describe in nine categories the depressed patients studied by the different authors, but, even so, he has been obviously compelled to include under the same heading – for example, endogenous depression – cases with different meanings for different authors. It has been repeatedly demonstrated that the present systems of diagnostic criteria for endogenous depression have a relatively small common variance. On the other hand, it is a well-known fact that the DSM-III does not include the category „neurotic depression“ (not to be confused with „depressive neurosis“), because in one study by Klerman and coworkers no agreement could be found on the diagnostic criteria implicitly used by American psychiatrists for that category. That we need clear and common diagnostic criteria for the subclasses of depression or mania is evident, and Angst has conclusively shown that many of the negative results obtained can be probably explained by the heterogeneous nature of the samples of patients, which lumped together under a generic term – such as depression – heterogeneous cases with different courses. I would like to quote an anecdote told by William Sargant about 30 years ago, although it concerns a slightly different subject, the demonstration in double-blind controlled studies of the statistically significant superiority of a psychotropic drug. Sargant remarked that in the eighteenth century there was a class of diseases known as the „fevers,“ which included in fact all of the infectious diseases whose common symptom was a high temperature. He suggested that if, at that time, a well-planned experiment had been made to demonstrate the therapeutic value of quinine, by taking two matched samples of „fever" patients, and by using quinine in one group and placebo in the controls, the difference would probably not have been significant, because the percentage of malaria patients was small and diluted in the group of „fevers." We are possibly with the present „affective disorders" in the same situation: depression corresponds possibly to the fevers of the eighteenth century and many of the negative results may be linked with our category of affective disorders.

It is true that we have made some progress. Professor Angst has repeatedly in his paper stressed the value of the distinction between bipolar and unipolar disorders, a change in classification for which he is responsible, and which has been considered by Kendell as the main progress made in the clinical study of the affective disorders since World War II. But there are many other unsolved questions, some of which I have briefly quoted, the definition of endogenous and of neurotic depression being the most obvious one. Angst has indicated the autonomy of bereavement, a fairly well-documented category. The introduction by the DSM-III of the „Major depressive episodes with mood incongruent psychotic symptoms" raises difficult questions, as well as the definition of „delusional depressions" and many others. Coming back to my discussion of the diagnostic criteria of affective disorders in general, I would like to stress that our efforts must be extended to the subcategories. Only if we reach some sort of agreement, can we hope to obtain results which, being comparable, can become significant.

If the definition of the cases, at the levels of the categories and of the subcategories, is the basic difficulty in all future studies of the course of the affective disorders, other problems have been raised by Angst.

He has rightly pointed out that older studies are interesting since, although they do have many drawbacks – for example, they are usually concerned with hospitalized patients, and the diagnostic criteria are not explicit – they deal with nontreated patients, and thus provide us with basic data on the natural course of the disease. Every research worker knows today that the extension of the therapy brings with it insurmountable difficulties by introducing uncontrollable bias.

The technique of retrospective studies, many of which have been quoted by Angst, is, as he rightly pointed out, very dangerous. I shall only refer in this context to two subjects: changes with time of the age of onset and of the frequency of depression. Recently the results of an American group were presented by Klerman. It was affirmed that, since the beginning of the century, the age of onset has decreased and the frequency increased. Although the authors claim to have taken every possible methodological precaution, the simple fact that the results are based on retrospective information makes the conclusions doubtful. Finally, I agree with Angst's statement that „Longitudinal population surveys with repeated measurements would be most important. Such studies require much time, money, and staff, but may turn out to be far more relevant and representative than any other work in the field."

I shall conclude this brief discussion by pointing out again to the high quality of Angst's paper. He has provided us in a clear and concise fashion with the essentials from an enormous literature. Although he has been able to extract some definitely established facts, he has made us aware of the many inadequacies of our knowledge and has suggested specific domains of research. We can of course differ with him on some minor points, and make them a subject for further discussion, but with his general conclusions we can only agree.

Genetic Aspects in Affective Disorders: Introductory Remarks

A. BERTELSEN

The main research methodologies in psychiatric genetics have been family studies, twin studies, and adoption strategies. Each of the methods has its limitations, but together they can provide evidence for genetical and environmental hypotheses.

Family Studies

The family studies are based on the Weinberg proband method and in representative samples they give lifetime morbid risk figures or expectancies for groups of relatives for comparison with the corresponding risk figures in the general population (Table 1).

Table 1. Expectancy (%) of affective disorders in family studies. (Data from Zerbin-Rüdin 1967)

	Expectancy (%)
Parents	7.4–23.4
Siblings	3.6–23.0
Children	8.4–24.1
Children of 2 manic-depressives	44 –74
Halfsiblings	1.4–16.7
Grandchildren	1.9– 3.3
First cousins	3.6

In manic-depressive disorders, family studies show expectancies among first-degree relatives of around 14% (range 4%–24%, Zerbin-Rüdin 1967). Expectancies for parents are almost equal to those for siblings and children. A female preponderance is observed in all groups of relatives, in accord with the general preponderance of females in affective disorders. In second-degree relatives, expectancies drop off to about one-third of the expectancies among first-degree relatives and in third-degree relatives to even less (Table 2).

Institute of Psychiatric Demography, Århus Psychiatric Hospital, DK-8240 Risskov

Depressive Illness: Prediction of Course and Outcome
Edited by T. Helgason and R. J. Daly

Table 2. Expectancy (%) of bipolar and unipolar illness in first-degree relatives (Gershon 1983)

	Bipolar	Unipolar
Bipolar probands	2.5–17.7	4.2–22.4
Unipolar probands	0.3– 4.1	5.9–17.5

Table 3. Dual mating studies: expectancy (%) of affective disorders in offspring of two parents with affective disorders

	Offspring > 15 years (*n*)	Expectancy (%)
Elsässer (1952; including Kahn and Schulz)	48	44
Lewis (1957)	22	58
Gershon et al. (1982)	28	74

Table 4. Pairwise concordance (%) in Manic-depressive twin series

	Monozygotic pairs		Dizygotic pairs	
	(*n*)	(%)	(*n*)	(%)
Luxenburger (1928)	3	67	13	0
Rosanoff et al. (1934)	23	70	67	16
Essen-Möller (1941)	8	25	3	0
Slater and Shields (1953)	8	50	30	24
Kallmann (1954)	27	93	55	24
Da Fonseca (1959)	21	71	39	38
Kringlen (1967)	6	33	20	0
Allen et al. (1974)	15	33	34	0
Bertelsen et al. (1977)	55	58	52	17
Kringlen (1980)	18	67	64	9

Heterogeneity has been suggested, dividing affective disorders into bipolar and unipolar illness. Relatives of bipolar probands have higher risk of bipolar illness and higher total risk of affective disorder than relatives of unipolar probands (Gershon 1983). The distinction is, however, far from complete. In the majority of studies there are more unipolars than bipolars among the relatives of bipolar probands, and bipolars also appear among the relatives of unipolar probands. Further heterogeneity has been suggested for both bipolar and unipolar illness but has not found uniform support (Table 3).

Studies of children of two affected parents, dual-mating studies, present a refinement of the family study design. Children of two manic-depressive parents have higher expectancies ranging from 44% to 74% in a recent study (Gershon et al. 1982). Dual-mating studies further permit a study of the interaction between genetic components of various psychiatric disorders (Table 4).

Twin Studies

In twin studies a higher concordance rate in monozygotic twins than in dizygotic twins is evidence of a genetic component. Monozygotic concordance of less than 100%, on the other hand, demonstrates the influence of environmental factors. Twin studies of manic-depressive psychosis have high monozygotic rates in some of the earlier studies, particularly in Kallmann's (1954) study. The studies have been criticized for selection bias with preferential ascertainment of concordant twins, overweight of severe cases, and use of loose diagnostic criteria with lack of blind assessment. This may apply to some of the earliest series based on hospital resident samples but not to the series of Slater and Shields (1953) and Da Fonseca (1959), which were based on consecutive samples. Kallmann unfortunately did not publish his case histories, but colleagues visiting and working in his department with access to his material, among others the Danish psychiatrist Borup Svendsen, have confirmed that Kallmann's diagnoses appeared quite reliable and were not based on a particularly wide concept; his amazingly high concordance may to some extent be explained by the inclusion of a high number of severe bipolar cases with high concordance.

The more recent studies have tried to make up for the shortcomings of the earlier studies and have managed to obtain more unselected and representative series based on twin and case registers. Some of the most recent studies, however, also show quite high concordance figures. The actual sizes of the concordance rates seem to depend more on the diagnostic concept and the strictness of the criteria for concordance applied in the individual series, and therefore the ratios between the monozygotic and dizygotic rates within the series are more interesting. All the twin studies show consistently higher monozygotic than dizygotic rates by a factor of 2 to 6 or more, indicating a strong genetic component. Supporting evidence comes from monozygotic pairs reared apart in which no shared family environment may contribute to the concordance. Pairs separated at an early age are few and only 12 manic-depressive pairs have been collected from the literature. Eight of the 12 pairs were concordant presenting the same concordance rate as the unseparated monozygotic twins in the series (Price 1968; Table 5).

The bipolar-unipolar distinction has been supported by a preponderance of bipolar/bipolar and unipolar/unipolar concordant monozygotic pairs (Table 6). On the other hand, the number of bipolar/unipolar concordant pairs confirms that a bipolar predisposition may manifest itself in a unipolar way only (Zerbin-Rüdin 1969; Bertelsen et al. 1977).

Table 5. Bipolar-unipolar concordance in monozygotic twins (Zerbin-Rüdin 1969; Bertelsen et al. 1977)

	Series	Casuistics
Both unipolar	20	13
Both bipolar	18	17
one unipolar, one bipolar	9	5

Table 6. Expectancy (%) in offspring of twins discordant for Manic-depressive disorder (Bertelsen 1985)

Parents	MZ pairs		DZ pairs		Half-siblings	
	(*n*)	(%)	(*n*)	(%)	(*n*)	(%)
Proband	47	10.5	74	17.1		
Co-twin	41	9.3	105	2.4	33	2.6

MZ, monozygotic; *DZ*, dizygotic.

Investigation of the risk among the offspring of affected and nonaffected twin partners presents a combination and refinement of the family and twin study method. In the Danish twin study, the expectancy among the children of the concordant monozygotic manic-depressive twins was similar to the expectancy among the children of their discordant partners, but highly different from the expectancy in the children of discordant dizygotic partners – which was of the same magnitude as for halfsiblings who also are second-degree relatives of the affected twins (Bertelsen 1985)

Adoption Strategies

The adoption strategies present a major advantage in the methodologies in psychiatric genetics, making it possible to demonstrate with certainty the importance of a genetic component. Adoption strategies have also been used in a few minor studies on affective disorders. Among the adoption studies two strategies should be distinguished. The adoptee's design and the adoptee's family study design (Table 7).

The adoptee's design applied by Cadoret (1978) investigates the prevalence of affective disorder in adopted-away children of parents with primary affective disorder compared to the prevalence in matched controls of adopted-away children of nonaffective parents, all reared by normal adoptive parents. The prevalence which should not be confused with morbid risk is clearly higher in the index adoptees, demonstrating the effect of a genetic component (Table 8).

Table 7. Adoptee's study design: affective disorders in adoptees of parents with affective disorders (Cadoret 1978)

Biological parents	Adoptees with affective disorders	
	(*n*)	Affected
Affective disorders	8	3
Other psychiatric disorders	75	4
No psychiatric disorders	43	4

Table 8. Adoptee's family study design: affective spectrum in parents of bipolar and normal adoptees (Mendlewicz and Rainer 1977)

	Biological parents	Adoptive parents
Index probands (29)	18	7
Control probands (22)	1	4
Nonadopted bipolar MD (31)	16	
Nonadopted poliomyelitis (20)	4	

MD, manic-depressive disorder.

The adoptee's family study design applied by Mendlewicz and Rainer (1977) investigates the prevalence of affective disorders in the biological and adoptive relatives of adoptees with bipolar illness compared to the relatives of matched normal control adoptees. The biological relatives showed a significantly higher prevalence of affective disorders than the adoptive relatives, giving confirming evidence of a genetic factor.

Linkage Analysis

Linkage analysis is the most powerful method for demonstration of genetic etiology. Psychiatric disorders with varying age of onset and possible lack of a major gene or with heterogeneity are, however, less likely to present linkage with a genetic marker, and the number of known genetic markers is still limited. In affective disorders some studies have presented evidence of linkage with color-blindness, with glucose-6-phosphate dehydrogenase deficiency, and with blood and HLA groups, but so far the findings seem to apply to subgroups of affective disorders only, indicating heterogeneity (Risch and Baron 1982). Recent advances in molecular biology have provided a technology for generating artificial genetic markers such as the DNA restriction fragment length polymorphisms for linkage analysis (Gusella et al. 1983), and this approach appears highly promising for future research in psychiatric genetics.

Mode of Transmission

The mode of transmission in affective disorders is still unknown. Some observations appear compatible with single major locus models and others with polygenic multifactorial models and a combined model with one specific gene in common and a number of modifying genes may be the most probable suggestion. Further progress will have to await the discovery of a stable characteristic of the genotype, a state-independent trait or biological indicator, which can be assessed in all carriers whether they are affected or not. Such major breakthrough may be expected from more fundamental research, possibly in relation to studies of individuals at high risk, whereas the traditional genetic research mainly will be able to contribute refined observations depending on advances in diagnostic validity and reliability.

Areas of Needed Research

The main areas for needed research will probably be those outlined above. At present it may be of value to initiate registration of informative families, including three or more generations, with collection of blood samples for future linkage studies using recombinant DNA techniques, which may be available in a few years.

References

Allen MG, Cohen S, Pollin W, Greenspan SI (1974) Affective illness in veteran twins. A diagnostic review. Am J Psychiatry 131:1234–1239

Bertelsen A (1985) A Danish twin study of manic-depressive disorders. In: Sakai T, Tsuboi T (eds) Genetic aspects of human behavior. Igaku-Shoin, Tokyo, New York, pp 97–102

Bertelsen A, Harvald B, Hauge M (1977) A Danish twin study of manic-depressive disorders. Br J Psychiatry 130:330–351

Cadoret RJ (1978) Evidence for genetic inheritance of primary affective disorder in adoptees. Am J Psychiatry 135:463–465

Da Fonseca AF (1959) Análise heredo-clinica das pertubações afectivas. (Estudo de 60 pares de gemeos e seus consanguineos). Imprensa Portuguesa, Porto

Elsässer G (1952) Die Nachkommen geisteskranker Elternpaare. Thieme, Stuttgart

Essen-Möller E (1941) Psychiatrische Untersuchungen an einer Serie von Zwillingen. Acta Psychiatr Neurolog Scand (Suppl 23)

Gershon E (1983) The genetics of affective disorders. In: Grinspoon L (ed) Psychiatry update, vol 2, American Psychiatric Press, Washington, DC, pp 434–457

Gershon ES, Hamovit J, Guroff JJ, Dibble E, Leckman JF, Sceery W, Targum SD, Nurnberger JI, Goldin LR, Bunney WE (1982) A family study of schizoaffective, bipolar I, bipolar II, unipolar, and normal control probands. Arch Gen Psychiatry 39:1157–1167

Gusella JF, Wexler NS, Conneally PM, Naylor SL, Anderson MA, Tanzi RE, Watkins PC, Ottina K, Wallace MR, Sakaguchi AY, Yong AB, Shoulson I, Bonilla E, Martin JB (1983) A polymorphic DNA marker genetically linked to Huntington's disease. Nature 306 234–238

Kallmann FJ (1954) Genetic principles in manic-depressive psychosis. In: Hoch P, Zubin J (eds) Depression. Grune and Stratton, New York, pp 1–24

Kringlen E (1967) Heredity and environment in the functional psychoses. Universitetsforlaget, Oslo

Kringlen E (1980) On the genetics and nosology of affective disorders. In: Achté K, Aalberg V, Lönnqvist J (eds) Psychopathology of depression, Proceedings of the Symposium of the Section of Clinical Psychopathology of the World Psychiatric Association 1979. Psychiatria Fennica Supplementum, pp 19–25

Lewis AJ (1957) The offspring of parents both mentally ill. Acta Genet Stati Med (Basel) 7:349–366

Luxenburger H (1928) Vorläufiger Bericht über psychiatrische Serienuntersuchungen an Zwillingen. Gesamte Neurolog Psychiatr 116:297–326

Mendlewicz J, Rainer JD (1977) Adoptive study supporting genetic transmission in manic-depressive illness. Nature 268:327–329

Price J (1968) The genetics of depressive behaviour. In: Coppen A, Walk A (eds) Recent developments in affective disorders, a symposium. Br J Psychiatry, Spec Publ 2

Risch N, Baron M (1982) X-linkage and genetic heterogeneity in bipolar-related major affective illness: re-analysis of linkage data. Ann Hum Genet 46:153–166

Rosanoff AJ, Handy LM, Plesset IR (1934) The etiology of manic-depressive syndromes with special reference to their occurrence in twins. Am J Psychiatry 91:725–762

Slater E, Shields J (1953) Psychotic and neurotic illness in twins. Medical Research Council Special Report Series No. 278. Her Majesty's Stationary Office, London

Zerbin-Rüdin E (1967) Endogene Psychosen. In: Becker PE (ed) Human-genetik, ein kurzes Handbuch, V/2. Thieme, Stuttgart

Zerbin-Rüdin E (1969) Zur Genetik der depressiven Erkrankungen. In: Hippius H, Selbach H (eds) Das depressive Syndrom. Urban und Schwarzenberg, Berlin, pp 37–56

Genetic Aspects in the Course and Outcome of Affective Disorders

E. SMERALDI

Introduction

Consistently, familial, twin, and adoption studies all suggest that genetic and environmental factors and their specific interactions are involved in the etiology of affective disorders. That genetic factors are involved has been demonstrated, but neither their nature nor their mode of action, nor their pattern of transmission have been defined. To do this, the specific biochemical pathogenetic mechanism must be identified, but since we do not yet have this particular piece of information, we must first identify genetic markers for affective disorders. Then the susceptible phenotype can be identified through some biological system that can supply information even when there are no behavioral manifestations, which indeed may require interaction of nongenetic, environmental, and social factors before they appear. For this reason, many subjects may be classified falsely as negative for the disease susceptibility. On the other hand, to study genetic linkage for complex non-Mendelian traits requires at least some information about the formal genetics of the hypothetical systems (the main locus) of disease susceptibility in the given population.

Therefore, studies of the segregation of affective disorders in families to identify marker loci are absolutely necessary. Unfortunately, even within these limits, the study of the genetics of affective disorders has run into unusual troubles: There are no clinical, biological, or pharmacological data to indicate whether or not the affective disorders are etiopathogenetically homogeneous, and the relevant genetic system whose segregation pattern we want to know may also not be unitary, even for a single clinical phenotype.

Family studies show that the lifetime risk of developing affective disorders is about 3.5 times greater for first-degree relatives of the probands than for the general population, but it is quite low in comparison with the risks for other inherited diseases. In clinical practice it is usual to meet both patients with negative family histories and those from families with a very high concentration of secondary cases, and we have as yet no biological or clinical parameters that clearly distinguish between these two forms.

Not even the application of multiple-threshold genetic models has enabled us to identify even one criterion around which to organize the genetic hetero-

Institute of Biomedical Sciences, St. Paul Clinical Psychiatry, Via A. di Rudini 8, I-20142 Milano

Depressive Illness: Prediction of Course and Outcome
Edited by T. Helgason and R. J. Daly

geneity of affective disorders. Usually the genetic models have been applied to the families of all affective patients, and this has not resulted in the exclusion of either of the genetic hypotheses tested, SML or MFP. It appears to be more promising to test the multiple threshold models on a population that might be more homogeneous, based on either clinical criteria, such as polarity (Smeraldi et al. 1981), or pharmacological criteria, such as response to lithium treatment (Smeraldi et al. 1984a). Unfortunately, neither of these criteria is completely reliable. The definition of polarity depends on the age of the subject and the number of episodes, which means that there may well occur manic phases later (Akiskal et al. 1983). In addition, some subjects classified as unipolar patients may have psychopathological conditions that do not share the specific susceptibility system for the recurrent affective disorders. The definition of "good responder" to lithium is also difficult, even if differences in bioavailability are overcome by monitoring serum lithium levels. The course of affective disorders is unpredictable, with some patients whose lack of relapses while on lithium may be due only to chance, whereas patients who experienced relapses have in fact a better outcome than the spontaneous outcome of the disease would have been. It is not really surprising that application of multiple threshold genetic models has not been very productive because they deal with disease rates in the groups of first-degree relatives and information related to segregation in each family (that is the genetic heterogeneity) is lost.

Genetic Heterogeneity

Let us assume that there is heterogeneity in genetic systems of transmission and talk about our current work as a possible example of how to deal with this heterogeneity. First, it was necessary to find and to refine some method for selection of subgroups of affective patients with a common genetic background, that is, patients whose susceptibility for these disorders depends on a single genetic mechanism. This was obtained by studying the genetic transmission of disease susceptibility for each family (including information about second-degree relatives). For each family we tested the liability for a single major locus transmission (Table 1), applying both dominant and recessive segregation models with sex-effect (Smeraldi et al. 1984b; Gasperini et al. 1987).

The log-likelihood ratio for the values obtained with both models, which indicates for each family the fit for the two genetic hypotheses, was calculated. Of course this ratio does not give any information about the genetic transmission of the illness, but it is useful for detecting those families with a similar genetic transmission of susceptibility. In fact, the focus of the analysis is shifted from the patients to the families and examines how the morbidity risk is distributed among them. A further advantage is that all this information can be expressed by a single numerical index. Figure 1 shows the observed distribution of frequencies of the ratios, obtained to see if we were dealing with one or more populations. The distribution of the ratios for our families clearly dif-

Table 1. Parametric sets applied in our segregation analyses

		Dominant model	Recessive model
Penetrance AA	Males	0	0
	Females	0	0
Penetrance Aa	Males	0.923	0
	Females	0.936	0.001
Penetrance aa	Males	1	0.908
	Females	1	0.987
q values	1st analysis	0.013	0.066
	2nd analysis	0.010	0.071

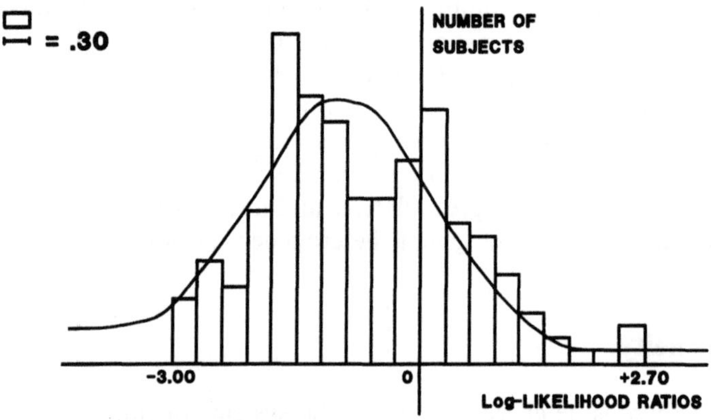

Fig. 1. Log-likelihood ratios distribution obtained by testing families according to the two alternative SML hypotheses with "q" values of 0.066 and 0.013

fers from normality, which could be obtained only in the case of a single genetic transmission for all affective disorders. Instead, we found at least two peaks of higher frequency, one around -1.65, the other around $+0.15$. These two peaks identify two groups of families with different segregation patterns. In each group, however, there may be a homogenous pattern of inheritance.

To separate our two populations better, we modified the values of allele frequency in the parametric set which have considerable effects on segregation analysis. We felt this correction to be acceptable since our aim was not to calculate the absolute values of genetic parameters, but only to separate families into more homoegeneous groups for testing neurochemical and pharmacological hypotheses. Calculation with these new values (Fig. 2) gave us two peaks of frequency that were further apart (median points, -1.65 and $+1.05$) and also revealed a third peak around zero, representing a group of families whose susceptibility system is probably different from the recessive vs dominant division.

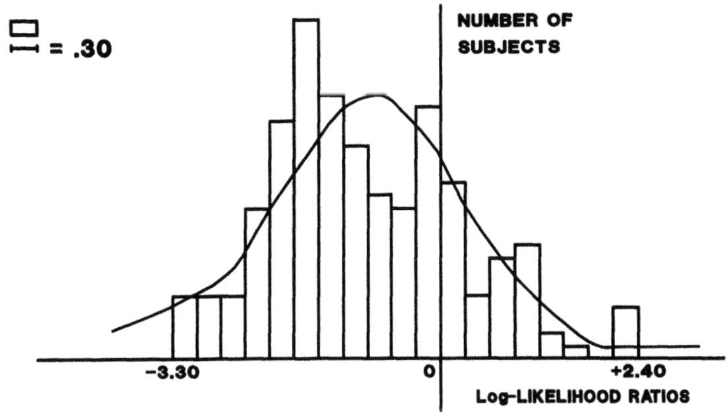

Fig. 2. Log-likelihood ratios distribution obtained by testing families according to the two alternative SML hypotheses with "q" values of 0.071 and 0.010

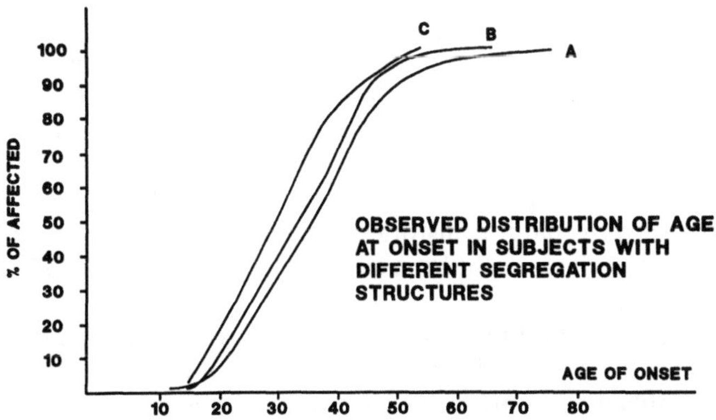

Fig. 3. Log-likelihood ratios

By this method we have obtained a reliable genetic dissection of affective disorders. By dealing with genetic heterogeneity, we have been able to identify three groups of families and therefore three groups of probands.

We then began to characterize the three groups of probands whose families had ratios near the three peaks clinically and pharmacologically.

First, we found that different familial structures condition different distributions of age at onset for the proband. As can be seen in Fig. 3, the A-type group of patients (to the left in Fig. 2) is characterized by later onset, the C-type group (to the right in Fig. 2) by an earlier age at onset, while the B-type group is intermediate. These differences are statistically significant.

Different familial structures are also related to different risks for suicide among secondary affective cases. In the families with ratio values consistent with dominant transmission (C type), there is a higher frequency of observed suicides among the relatives than in families with types A plus B ratios (8/41 vs 13/117). This difference might be associated with a monoaminergic abnormality. Van Praag (1982) has reported that the suicide rate was higher in depressive patients with low post-probenecid CSF 5-HIAA responses than in a normoserotoninergic subgroup. However, serotonin abnormalities are not found in all subjects with affective disorders, but only in a subgroup in which it appears to be a true susceptibility factor because it can be demonstrated whether or not the subject is clinically in depression. This subgroup may be the one that we have differentiated in our genetic studies as group C. This is supported by the observation (Van Praag and De Haan 1979; Sedvall et al. 1980) that the frequency of depression in families of probands with 5-HT disorder is greater than in families of other affective patients. Our group C families contain more secondary cases than those of groups A and B.

An interesting observation is that among the probands from A-type families there was the lowest frequency of subjects treated with lithium salts (45% vs 65% of the other groups), even though all the other variables that are usually taken into account in the clinical lithium studies turned out to be randomly distributed among groups, namely the duration of illness, the sex of the proband, and, most surprisingly, the polarity of the disease. One possibility that still needs to be tested is that probands with A-type families, that is, with lower genetic loads, also have natural histories of the disease with a lower spontaneous relapsing rate, which might have caused many of them not to be treated preventively with lithium.

However, when treated with lithium, patients in the three groups did not differ in the rates of relapse. We must keep in mind that, methodologically, it is rather difficult to reliably define patients as good or poor responders during long-term lithium treatment, because of possible differences in the spontaneous relapsing rates.

Discussion

Once genetic heterogeneity has been accepted, the idea should stimulate investigation into its biological meaning. According to recent data reported by Prusoff et al. (1985), we felt that useful information should be obtained, for example, by studying the correlation between family structures of susceptibility and the responses of their probands to antidepressant drugs. We could find no associations when antidepressant drugs were considered as a whole. However, when we broke down our data, we found they did suggest possible relations with the major categories of drugs, for example, those acting on the serotoninergic system. This possibility has to be further investigated in light of the hypothesis we mentioned before, when speaking of family clusters with high suicide rates.

Genetic heterogeneity of affective disorders could also explain the conflicting results obtained in the studies of association and linkage of HLA and affective disorders. In the Italian population we have detected an excess of HLA similarities in doubly affected siblings and a lack of similarities in discordant siblings (Smeraldi and Bellodi 1981). When two or more siblings are affected, the segregation of HLA haplotypes is no longer completely independent (that is 25%, 50%, 25%), but is deviated by the linkage between the HLA complex and the disease susceptibility gene. From our data, this main locus was mapped on the short arm of chromosome 6 at 0.125 recombinant units from the HLA complex. Weitkamp et al. (1981) and Kidd (1982) reported similar results, whereas Goldin et al. (1982) and Suarez and Reich (1984) were not able to demonstrate any relationship between HLA and major affective disorders. We are not greatly impressed by this discrepancy. The inconsistency of the results could well result from analysis of data which did not take into account any genetic heterogeneity of the illness, but analysed it as a single entity. In other words, all the discrepancies found could be due merely to different patient ascertainment. Different patient samples might well contain different proportions of pedigrees with different segregation patterns, either by chance or because of differences in the allele frequencies in the populations tested.

It is very common to find the same situation when other biological characteristics that are reported to be genetic markers of the disorder or to be associated with it are studied, for instance, imipramine binding sites in platelets, platelet MAO activities, and muscarinic receptor density. My feeling is that the usefulness of such studies could be greatly enhanced if the heterogeneity of affective disorders were included in the model.

Conclusion

Let me attempt to derive a more general conclusion. In genetic studies of psychiatric disorders we work with the segregation of disease susceptibility not with the segregation of the disorder itself. The route from the gene to the phenotype is quite complex. Even if a single genotype does underly the disease, we can observe clinical entities which differ greatly in severity, which gives a clinical spectrum with several intermediate phenotypes. In our studies, we employed only diagnoses narrowly defined according to the DSM-III first axis for both the probands and the secondary cases. It may be sensitivity would be increased by extending the analysis to patients with second axis diagnoses, that is, with personality disorders, some subgroups of alcoholism, and, possibly, also disorders still separated from affective disorders according to clinical criteria but similar psychopharmacologically, such as panic attacks. Perhaps the frequencies of these other diagnoses differ in families of the different types, as, for example, the frequency of suicide does, and this would be helpful for accentuating differences in segregation.

Finally, when dealing with the genetics of affective disorders, we must also consider the possible consequences of other well-known variables, such as assortative mating effects (Negri et al. 1981) and the changes in penetration from one generation to another. Both of these variables are generally accepted to be involved, but have always been studied without including the heterogeneity of the affective disorders in the analysis, and we do not know at present how they may separate out in different types of families.

In conclusion, new approaches and strategies have been attempted by applying modern genetic techniques and hypotheses to the studies of affective disorders. Much helpful information has been obtained. However, major basic problems still prevent us from taking the greatest possible advantage of such studies: they are mainly connected to sample selection and to the definition of phenotype and are quite difficult to cope with, since they are strictly dependent on the heterogeneity itself of the disorder.

References

Akiskal HS, Walker P, Puzantian VR et al. (1983) Bipolar outcome in the course of depressive illness – phenomenologic, familial and pharmacologic predictors. J Affective Disord 5:115

Gasperini M, Orsini A, Bussoleni L et al. (1987) Genetic approach to the study of heterogeneity of affective disorders. J Affective Disord 12:105

Goldin RL, Clerget-Darpoux F, Gershon ES (1982) Relationship of HLA to major affective disorder not supported. Psychiatry Res 7:29

Kidd KK (1982) Genetic linkage markers in the study of psychiatric disorders. In: E Usdin, I Hani (eds) Biological markers in psychiatry and neurology. Pergamon, Oxford, pp 459

Negri F, Melica AM, Zuliani R et al. (1981) Genetic implication in assortative mating of affective disorders. Br J Psychiatry 138:236

Prusoff BA, Weissman MM, Merikangas KR et al. (1985) Drug response as a predictor of transmission of non-bipolar major depression within families. J Affective Disord 8:171

Sedvall G, Fyro B, Gulberg B et al. (1980) Relationships in healthy volunteers between concentration of monoamine metabolites in cerebrospinal fluid and family history of psychiatric morbidity. Br J Psychiatry 136:366

Smeraldi E, Bellodi L (1981) Possible linkage between primary affective disorders susceptibility locus and HLA haplotypes. Am J Psychiatry 138:1232

Smeraldi E, Negri F, Heimbuch RC, Kidd KK (1981) Familial patterns and possible modes of inheritance of primary affective disorders. J Affective Disord 3:173

Smeraldi E, Petroccione A, Gasperini M et al. (1984 a) Outcomes on lithium treatment as a tool for genetic studies in affective disorders. J Affective Disord 6:139

Smeraldi E, Petroccione A, Gasperini M et al. (1984 b) The search for genetic homogeneity in affective disorders. J Affective Disord 7:99

Suarez BK, Reich T (1984) HLA and major affective disorders. Arch Gen Psychiatry 41:22

Van Praag HM (1982) Depression, suicide and the metabolism of serotonin in the brain. J Affective Disord 4:275–290

Van Praag HM, De Haan S (1979) Central serotonin metabolism and frequency of depression. Psychiatry Res 1:219

Weitkamp LR, Stancer HC, Persad E et al. (1981) Depressive disorders and HLA: a gene on chromosome 6 that can affect behavior. N Engl J Med 305:1301

Psychosocial Aspects of Course and Outcome in Depressive Illness

H. KATSCHNIG and D. O. NUTZINGER

Introduction

"Psychosocial" is an umbrella term with very little meaning in itself. It is, therefore, necessary to be as specific as possible when "psychosocial" factors are discussed in relation to research on the course of depressive disorders. Personality factors, the classical social variables of sex, social class, or marital status, as well as more complex phenomena, such as life events, social network, or social support, all can be subsumed under the label "psychosocial."

In the field of "psychosocial" factors we are far away from being able to deal with the vast amount of knowledge that Angst has presented in his paper (this volume) using such clinical variables as switch from depressive to manic episode, frequency of episodes, recovery, and relapse rate. The lack of agreed-upon definitions of specific variables, which already besets clinical research – clinical outcome criteria, for example, differ from one study to another – especially hampers psychosocial research.

Before discussing some methodological issues needing closer attention in future research, some existing studies concerning course and outcome of depressive illness in relation to psychosocial variables will be briefly discussed. In order to do this, a schematic framework for the possible place of psychosocial factors in such studies is provided.

The Place of Psychosocial Factors in Course and Outcome Studies

When analyzing the role of psychosocial factors in the course and outcome of depression, it is useful to be aware of the logical place of psychosocial factors in possible study designs. This is best achieved by use of a diagram showing the possible roles of both "psychosocial factors" and "nonpsychosocial factors" – the latter comprising psychopathological and biological variables – at different stages of the development of the disorder.

Psychiatrische Universitätsklinik, Währinger Gürtel 18–20, A-1090 Vienna

Four such stages are distinguished: (a) the course before the index episode, (b) the index episode itself, (c) the course between the index episode and the follow-up evaluation, and, finally, (d) the follow-up or outcome assessment. All variables – both the psychosocial and nonpsychosocial ones – can be and are, in fact, used both as predictor and as predicted variables depending on the design of the study. This is illustrated by the bars on the left side of Fig. 1.

Those psychosocial factors exerting their influence before and at the onset of the index episode – such as personality factors or life events precipitating the index episode – can be used to predict variables of the index episode (such as its duration), as well as psychosocial and nonpsychosocial course and outcome characteristics (A). Characteristics of the index episode such as its length or specific symptoms may be used as predictor variables for course and outcome (B). Finally, events occurring after the index episodes may modify the course of the disorder and determine outcome variables (C).

It has to be kept in mind that all kinds of "cross predictions" are possible, i.e., psychosocial variables may not only predict psychosocial but also nonpsychosocial variables, and nonpsychosocial variables may determine both nonpsychosocial and psychosocial outcome criteria. Examples are shown in Fig. 2. For example, brain trauma before the index episode may predict the number of relapses (1); severity of symptoms at the index episode may be related to poor psychosocial adjustment at follow-up (2). Precipitating life events at the onset of the index episode may be related to a shortened duration of the index episode (3) and, finally, life events during the follow-up period may be connected with poor psychosocial outcome (4). All other types of relationships are, of course, conceivable and it seems useful to analyse a given study by use of this diagram to become aware of the nature of the question which can or cannot be answered by the design of the study.

Apart from these possible relationships between predictor and predicted variables, the actual way of how and when data are collected is especially relevant for studying psychosocial variables. Whether a study is retrospective (Fig. 3) or prospective (Fig. 4) may matter a lot for the quality of the results, since exclusive retrospective collection of psychosocial data at the time of the follow-up evaluation may easily create spurious relationships (see below; Monroe and Steiner 1986). A prospective design with repeated evaluations at the index episode and at later stages would help to reduce such "contamination" but is, of course, much more expensive and therefore rarely applied.

We have identified seven typical questions in relation to psychosocial variables and the course and outcome of depressive illness, which have so far been addressed by researchers. These questions are not necessarily clearly separated from each other but rather represent some typical foci of interest in present research. The examples are only intended to illustrate these questions and not to give any definite answers, since differences in study design and methodology prevent such definite conclusions. Therefore these questions point to existing gaps in our knowledge.

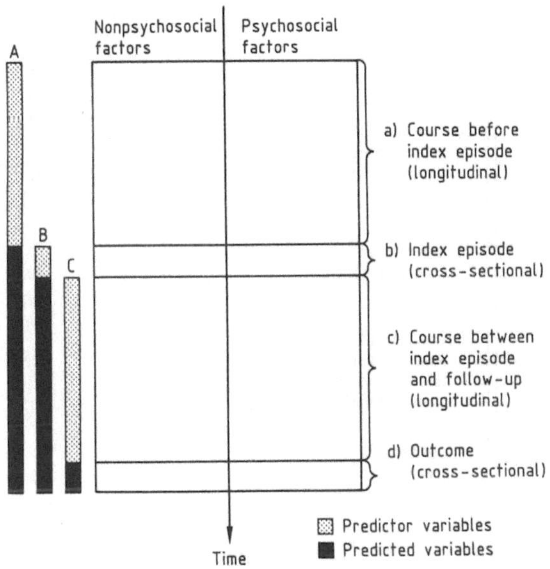

Fig. 1. Nonpsychosocial and psychosocial factors as predictor and predicted variables 1; *A, B, C,* see text

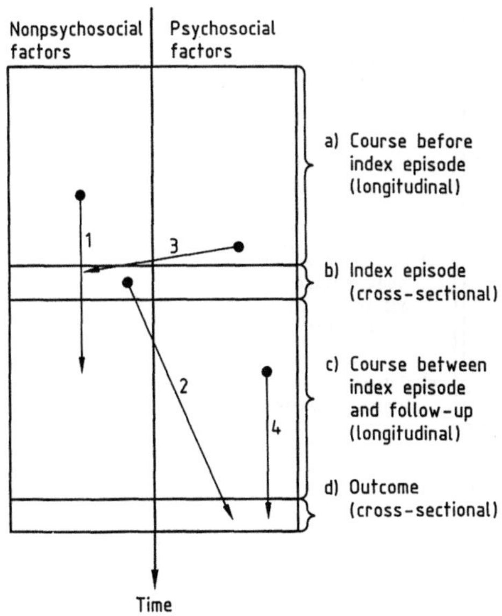

Fig. 2. Nonpsychosocial and psychosocial factors as predictor and predicted variables 2; *1, 2, 3, 4,* see text

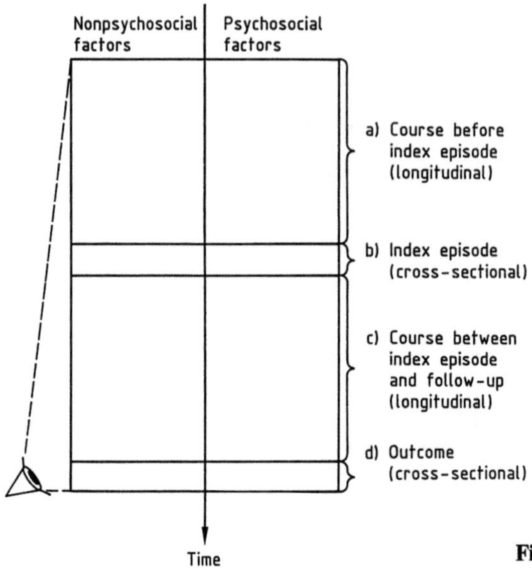

Fig. 3. Retrospective research design

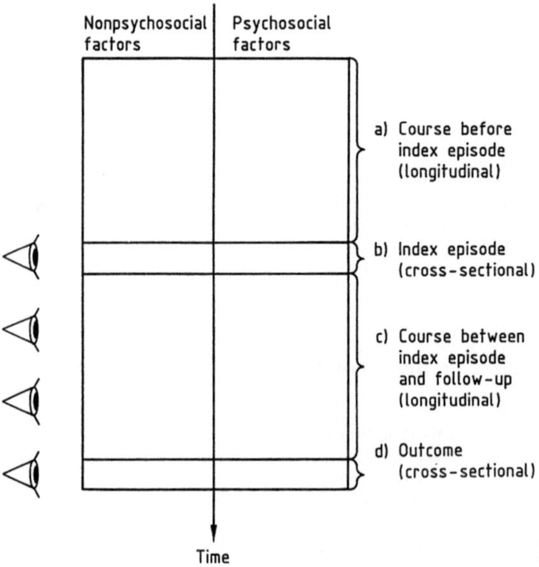

Fig. 4. Prospective research design

Type 1: Premorbid Personality as a Predictor Variable

In addition to the long-standing question of whether persons suffering from depressive or manic-depressive illness have specific premorbid personality traits (Katschnig et al. 1983, p 396 ff.), some studies have explicitly addressed the possible influence of different premorbid personality traits on course and outcome of depression. Figure 5 shows that a wide variety of possible influences of premorbid personality exist.

As early as 1942 Rennie observed that an "outgoing make-up" of the personality was a strong predictor for a good outcome in manic-depressive psychosis. Weissman et al. (1978), Katschnig and Egger-Zeidner (1985), and Hirschfeld et al. (1986) found a high predictive power for some personality variables (e.g., for neuroticism which predicts bad outcome), but they could not establish a relationship between most other psychosocial variables and outcome measures. In contrast, Wittchen and von Zerssen (1988) found that personality variables were relatively unimportant for outcome in comparison with psychopathological variables and social support measures. In the Newcastle study (Kay et al. 1969), the personality dimension "narrow interests" was related to an unfavorable course.

The measurement of personality traits is a complex issue. It is quite reasonable to assume that personality, social support, life events, and psychopathological phenomena are connected with each other (Monroe and Steiner 1986). Especially in retrospective research designs it may prove very difficult to disentangle these different measures (see below).

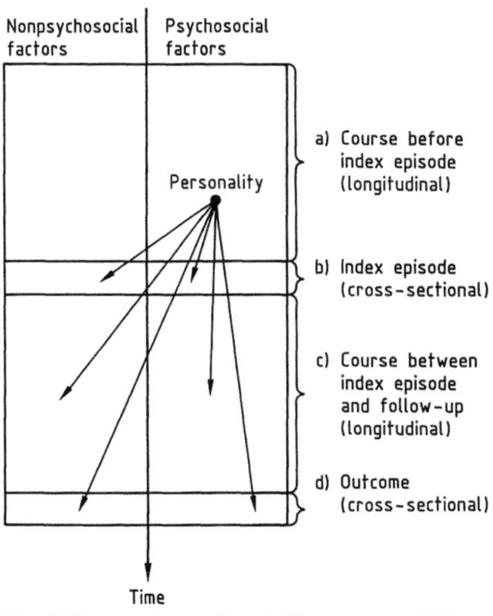

Fig. 5. Research question 1: Does premorbid personality influence the course and outcome of depressive disorders?

Type 2: Sociodemographic Variables and Premorbid Psychosocial Adjustment as Predictor Variables

Age, sex, marital status, and other demographic variables – in contrast to personality variables – can be easily collected at the time of the index episode. Some of these variables, such as marital status or professional activities, are sometimes regarded as representing a measure for social ajustment. Possible questions are shown in Fig. 6.

A typical question in this field is the relationship between age at onset and course. Angst (this volume) has analysed the literature and concluded that late age of onset is clearly correlated with more relapses. Katschnig and Egger-Zeidner (1985) found no relationship between both age at onset and at admission and the development of a chronic course or the suicide rate, whereas Kay et al. (1969) in a 5- to 7-year follow-up study identified increased age as a good prognostic factor. The short-term outcome measured as the length of the episode is worse with increased age and is not influenced by sex, as was noted in a review of the literature by Bebbington (1982). As far as sex is concerned, several studies suggest that males have a better outcome (e.g., Kerr et al. 1972). Marital status was not found to be important by Keller and Shapiro (1981), a result which is identical with findings by Weissman et al. (1978), Goering et al. (1983), and Katschnig and Egger-Zeidner (1985). However, some earlier studies (Burke et al. 1967; Clum 1966) have indicated a positive influence of being married.

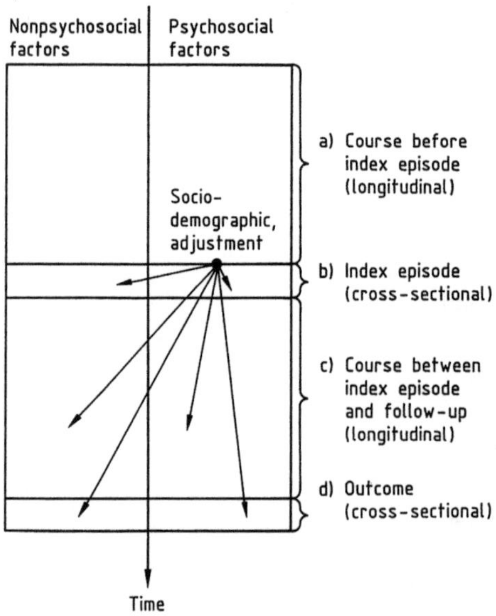

Fig. 6. Research question 2: Do premorbid psychosocial adjustment and socio-demographic variables influence the course and outcome of depressive disorders?

These classical social category variables have clear limitations and should be supplemented by more subtle measures, describing, e.g., the quality of a relationship and the perception of it (see below), or work satisfaction in addition to objective working conditions. Henderson et al. (1980) have developed a research instrument, the "Interview Schedule of Social Interaction," which covers also these more subtle aspects of social variables. For example, Katschnig and Egger-Zeidner (1985) found high work satisfaction at the index episode predictive of a good prognosis in depression, while the simple categorical variable social class and similar measures were insignificant for outcome.

Here again, as in studies on premorbid personality, the interrelationships between several variables will have to be studied, including the subdivision into clinical subtypes, before conclusive evidence about predictors becomes available.

Type 3: Psychosocial Precipitants of the Index Episode as Predictor Variables

Kraepelin (1909) was quite open to the issue that some depressive and even some manic episodes were triggered by severely threatening events, such as the death of a loved one or one's own physical disease. However, he noted that among 49 such cases, 24 further episodes were observed which were not triggered by life stress and he puts forward the modern statistical issue of chance agreement as one possibility of explaining the coincidence of life stress and

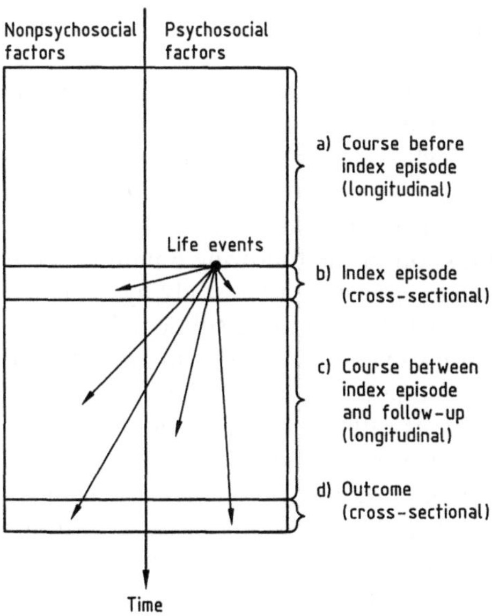

Fig. 7. Research question 3: Are psychosocial precipitants of the index episode of any importance for the prognosis of depressive disorders?

episode onset. Scandinavian psychiatrists (Wimmer 1916; Strömgren 1974) have even created a specific nosological concept, that of "reactive psychoses," which are caused by "mental traumata" and are also characterized by the "predominant tendency... to recovery and, more specifically, that they never end in deterioration" (Strömgren 1974; Fig. 7).

In an early study, Swift (1907–1908) found that "exciting emotional causes" correlated with good prognosis. In 1942 Rennie, remarking that 80% of his patients had some reactive aspects at the index episode, found that reactivity did not matter for outcome. Endicott and Spitzer (1979) found no difference in outcome between situational and nonsituational depressions according to the Research Diagnostic Criteria (RDC), and Copeland (1984) replicated this negative finding. In the Vienna study, life events did not prove to be of any prognostic importance either for the development of chronicity or for suicide. In the Newcastle study, bereavement was favorable but any other "psychogenesis" was unfavorable for outcome (Kay et al. 1969). Monroe et al. (1985) in a therapeutic trial, found a favorable influence of precipitating life events on outcome, but only for the endogenous and not the nonendogenous subtype of depression.

The measurement of life stress is, again, a complex issue and its problems will be discussed below (see also Katschnig 1986).

Type 4: Social Network and Social Support as Predictor Variables

Intuitively the answer to the question of whether social support is connected with prognosis seems to be clear, i.e., it favors a good prognosis. Several studies indicate that this might, in fact, be the case (Fig. 8).

Surtees (1980) found a clear-cut influence of "social support" in the sense of preventing a reoccurrence of despressive symptoms in those persons who had a high "level of residual adversity," whom he studied over a 7-month period. Goering et al. (1983) confirmed this in a sample of 87 discharged women who had been treated for "nonpsychotic disorders"; the only significant factor distinguishing those who had a readmission in the following 6 months from those not readmitted was "lack of social support." In the study by Wittchen and von Zerssen (1988) social support measured by more subtle indices such as stable relationship with a partner, intimacy, and the like, also proved to be of positive influence. Henderson (1984), due to his results in a longitudinal community study in Canberra, Australia, is rather sceptical about the role of social support in the prevention of onset of depression; however, he admits that social support may, in fact, have an important effect on the course of psychiatric disorders. Kerr et al. (1972) showed that of several measures used for premorbid social adaptation, only marital disharmony was significantly related to poor prognosis, and Merikangas et al. (1983) in their study on married couples with a depressed partner demonstrated a significant effect on maladjustment at outcome, if the other partner was also depressed.

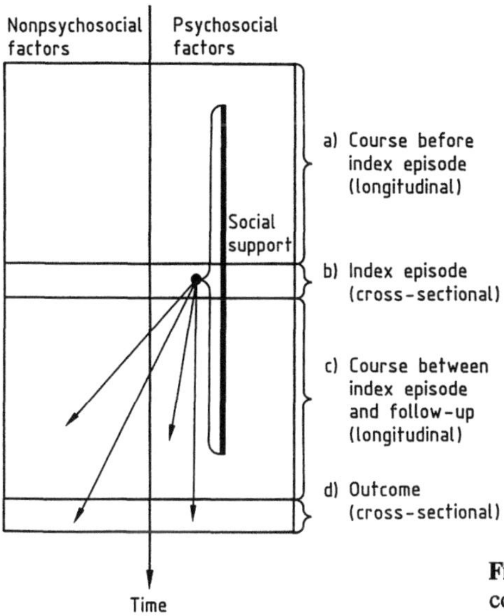

Fig. 8. Research question 4: Is social support connected with a better prognosis?

The problems with measuring social support are discussed below. One of them is shown in Fig. 8: it is not always clear which point in time the social support measure refers to.

Type 5: Diagnostic Subclassification ("Neurotic" Vs "Endogenous") as Predictor Variables

The "endogenous/neurotic" issue is a complex one and should, in fact, be considered when studying any of the other questions discussed in this paper, since in many definitions of the nonendogenous subtype psychosocial factors are included (see Katschnig et al. 1986a; Fig. 9).

There are only a few studies which explicitly address the question of a different outcome for different depressive subtypes. While Kay et al. (1969) in a 5- to 7-year follow-up and Paykel et al. (1974) in a 10-month longitudinal study found a better clinical (but not social) outcome for endogenous than for neurotic depression, Endicott and Spitzer (1979), using the Research Diagnostic Criteria for "endogenous" and "nonendogenous" found the reverse to be the case in a 2-year follow-up study. Equally, Copeland (1983) found a worse prognosis for psychotic than for neurotic patients in a 5-year follow-up. In the study by Katschnig et al. (1986b), the endogenous/neurotic subdivision – according to a number of different diagnostic criteria – did not show any significant difference in terms of chronicity or suicide rate during a 2-year follow-up period. It is quite clear that the definition of the study population is decisive for comparability and we will come back to this issue below.

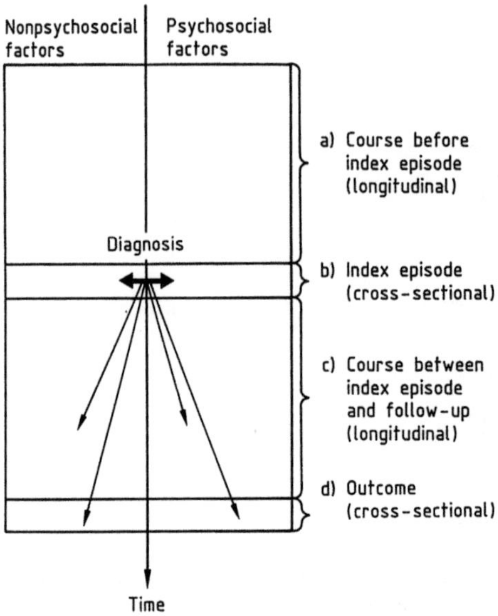

Fig. 9. Research question 5: Is the diagnostic subclassification into a "neurotic" and an "endogenous" type of depression important for course and outcome?

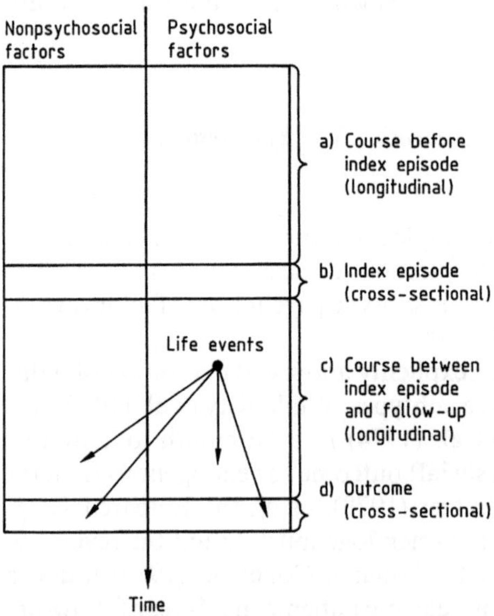

Fig. 10. Research question 6: Do psychosocial changes in a person's life occurring after the index episode and during the follow-up time influence course and outcome?

Type 6: Psychosocial Influences After the Index Episode as Predictor Variables

This is clearly a neglected area. Not only has the influence of therapy in long-term outcome studies been largely neglected so far, but also the possible occurrence of stressors between the index episode and the outcome evaluation has been largely neglected. Figure 10 illustrates this study design.

A few studies have, nevertheless, been carried out. Klerman (1980) and Bothwell and Weissman (1977) could demonstrate that the relapse rate was raised in those depressive patients who, despite the remission of the index episode, experienced life changes, especially interpersonal conflicts, during the follow-up period. Wittchen and von Zerssen (1988) found similar results, which they could differentiate according to diagnostic class: patients with affective psychosis had more loss events, more undesirable events, and also more events which were classed as subjectively more stressing. Positive events did not play any role for outcome in affective psychosis, while in neurotic depression the number of positive events was significantly higher in those patients with a better outcome than in those with a worse outcome. Tennant et al. (1981 a) demonstrated that neurotic disturbances which occurred after threatening life events improved considerably through so-called "neutralizing life events" (inside 1 month). Brown et al. (1988) could show in a study carried out in Islington/London on over 400 working-class women with children that in 60% of remissions of depression, the remission was the consequence of a positive event ending a long-term difficulty.

Type 7: Psychosocial Variables as Outcome Criteria

The previously discussed types of questions place psychosocial variables in the position of a predictor variable. It is frequently overlooked that psychosocial variables can also be used as outcome measures. Usually in psychiatric follow-up studies, clinical outcome measures – such as number of relapses, development of chronicity, time in hospital, etc. – prevail. Sometimes a mixture of clinical and social functioning variables is used which are combined into outcome indices. For instance, Bond and Braceland (1937) in their 5-year follow-up study on over 200 manic-depressed and melancholic patients used as a definition of recovery that patients had become "healthy and economically valuable." Equally, Hastings (1958) designed five outcome measures which were mixtures between clinical measures, such as time in hospital, and an evaluation of social adjustment. Shobe and Brion (1971) used a composite index including an assessment whether the person was "able to work and function socially" in addition to the number of episodes and time in hospital (Fig. 11).

The practice of constructing combined social and clinical outcome measures contrasts clearly with a finding by Weissman et al. (1974) showing a differential effect of drugs and psychotherapy on psychopathology and social ad-

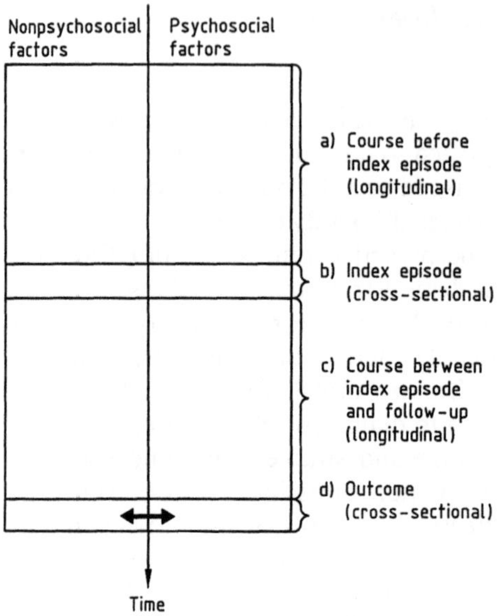

Fig. 11. Research question 7: Are social and clinical outcomes correlated?

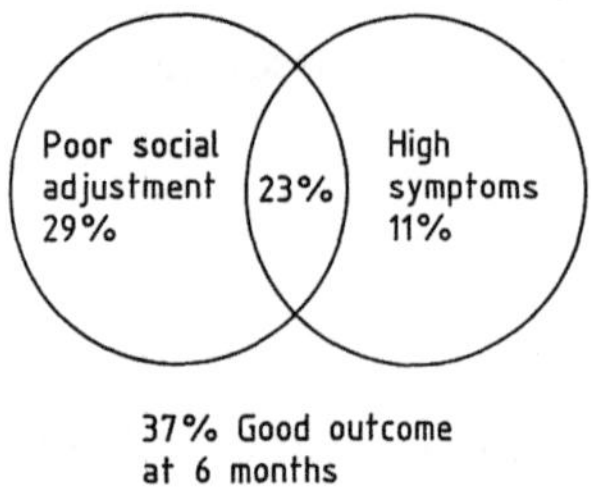

Fig. 12. Relationship between social adjustment and symptoms as outcome measures for 87 neurotic women (Goering et al. 1983)

justment. In a study by Merikangas et al. (1983), clinical course and outcome were not correlated with psychosocial outcome in married depressed patients. If the spouse of the patient was also depressed, significant maladjustment was measured after 1 to 3 years of follow-up (e.g., a divorce rate of 27% as opposed to 4% in depressed patients without a depressed spouse); however, relapse rate and symptomatology did not differ in the two groups. Finally, Goering et al. (1983) in a 6-month follow-up study of discharged depressed women showed a very low correlation between a high level of symptoms and "poor social adjustment." The authors have put their results into a very telling diagram (Fig. 12).

These results suggest the necessity of evaluating clinical outcome criteria and social adjustment separately by use of a multiaxial data collection system.

It goes without saying that, whenever social variables are used to measure outcome the studies must be controlled for the status of these variables at the index episode.

Some Methodological Issues Needing Closer Attention in Future Research

These few examples of answers to possible questions demonstrate how far away we are from a coherent body of knowledge as far as the influence of social factors on course and outcome of depression is concerned. The reason for these discrepancies is, as always and still in psychiatry, the different research designs and methodologies used in different research projects. These differences are also relevant for the clinicial studies quoted by Angst. Differences in diagnosing and selecting a study population, differences in the length of the follow-up period, differences in the course and outcome criteria chosen are only a few of these more general issues. When psychosocial factors are studied the lack of standardization of collecting these variables is an additional handicap.

The second part of this paper concentrates on some design and methodological issues which should receive more attention in future research. Three issues will be discussed: the selection of an appropriate model for studying social factors in relation to course and outcome; study design problems (including the definition of the study population); and, finally, problems with methods for measuring psychosocial variables.

The Selection of an Appropriate Model for Studying Social Factors in Course and Outcome

Strauss et al. (1985) have pointed out that traditional longitudinal research in psychiatry relies on a "natural history" model with its concept of a predetermined outcome which can be checked at a cross-sectional examination at follow-up. Such an approach is both cheaper and less cumbersome than "follow-along" studies, which try to accompany the patient and draw a picture of the course of the disorder and the possible external influences on it. If a fuller and undistorted view of both the course of depression and the outcome is to be obtained, the development between the index episode and outcome assessment cannot be disregarded. Discrepancies in results of outcome studies might be explained by the neglect of such intervening factors. This would mean a change in research paradigm from a "natural history" to a "vulnerability-stress" model, and even to an "interactive developmental" paradigm (Strauss et al. 1985).

Natural History Model

In this model nonpsychosocial factors, known for the time before or at the index episode should predict course and outcome. Figure 13 shows the assumptions of this "natural history model" of psychiatric disorders.

Basically, according to this model it should be possible to predict from psychiatric history and from cross-sectional phenomenological data such course and outcome criteria as number of subsequent episodes, duration and type of episode. However, the Kraepelinian model of psychiatric disease entities, each characterized by a specific etiology, a specific syndrome, and a specific course, has not been proven to date for a larger proportion of functional mental disorders. Variations in course and outcome of mental disorders are still substantial and have not yet been explained by nonpsychosocial factors alone.

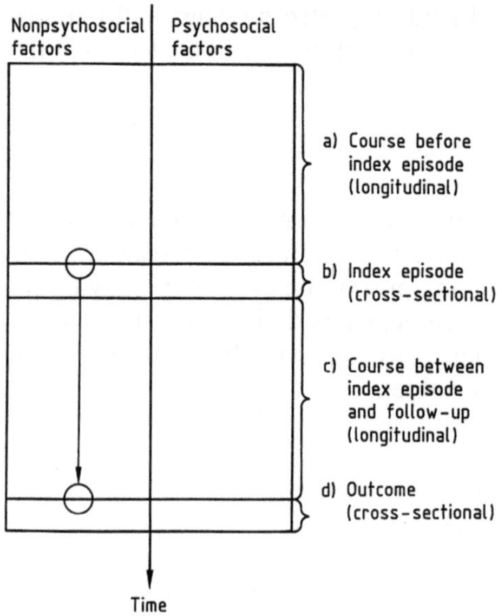

Fig. 13. Natural history model

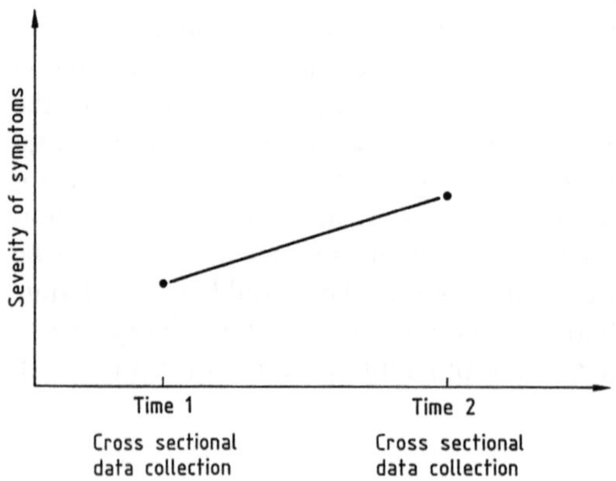

Fig. 14. Outcome study

When the natural history model is used, frequently a simple cross-sectional approach is applied, comparing the status at the index episode with the status at follow-up, i.e., a simple outcome study is carried out (Fig. 14).

Vulnerability-Stress Model

A vulnerability-stress model may be more appropriate to describe the *course* of depressive disorders, since it allows for later influences – stressors – to change the course. Such a "vulnerability-stress" model has already been in use at the time of Kraepelin for explaining the etiology of infectious diseases, it is only necessary to extend its scope from a mere etiological concept to a longitudinal course concept (Fig. 15).

The epidemiological triad of "host," "agent," and "environment" clearly emphasizes all three necessary elements to predict the outbreak of an infectious disease. For psychiatric disorders, this model has been adopted by several research workers (e.g., Brown and Harris 1978). If this model is extended to the course of the disorder, it accomodates some studies already cited – which show that adverse life events have a negative influence on the course of depression (Bothwell and Weissman 1977; Klerman 1980; Wittchen and von Zerssen 1988). More subtle analyses are, however, necessary, if the relatonship between such adverse life events and psychopathology during the course of depression is to be understood. Both the occurrence of life events and the course of symptomatology have to be recorded precisely in such studies in order to sort out

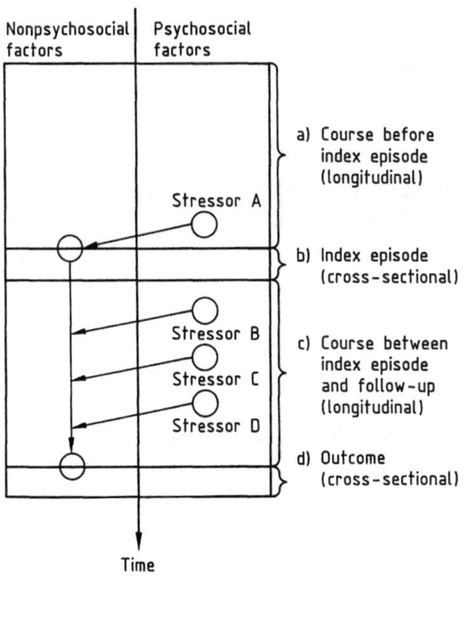

Fig. 15. Vulnerability stress model

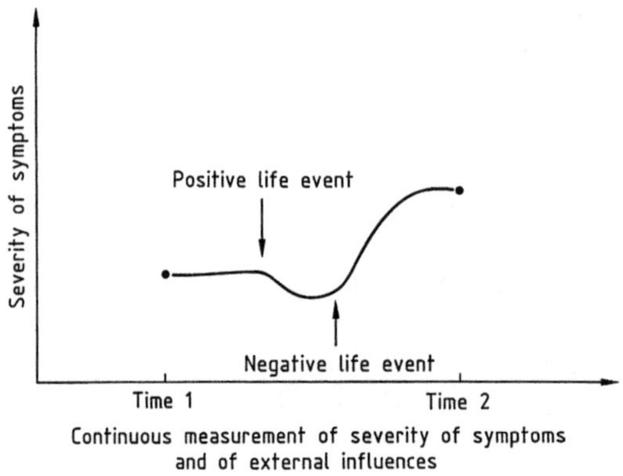

Fig. 16. Course study

cause and effect. We are currently on the way to analysing such data in our own research project.

While the same amount of psychopathology may be measured both in a cross-sectional outcome and a longitudinal course study for time 1 and time 2, respectively, and only a straight line is drawn between the two points in an outcome study (follow-up study; see Fig. 14), a course study (follow-along study) may reveal many details as shown in Fig. 16. Not only the changing course, but also possible psychosocial reasons for these changes can thus become apparent.

The "vulnerability-stress" model can be generalized to a "vulnerability-external influence" model, in order to incorporate also positive influences, such as naturally occurring positive life events and therapeutic interventions. Agras et al. (1972) have pointed out that the remission of phobia, especially in childhood, occurs naturally through the exposition of the child to the phobic stimulus, thus mirroring the processes which occur in behavior therapy. What looks like a spontaneous remission may simply be the consequence of some positively experienced event which remains unnoticed by the researchers. It is difficult to pick up therapeutic interventions in a naturalistic follow-up study, but it may be very important in order to explain individual changes in the course. A frequent reason for relapse missed in outcome studies is stopping medication (which in turn may depend on some environmental changes of the indvidual; see below).

Interactive Developmental Model

Strauss et al. (1985) have suggested a model which goes beyond the vulnerability-stress model, which they call an "interactive developmental model." In this model the more realistic assumption is implied that it is not only independent external influences which matter, but that the individual himself creates his environment and may thus be responsible for the occurrence of adverse,

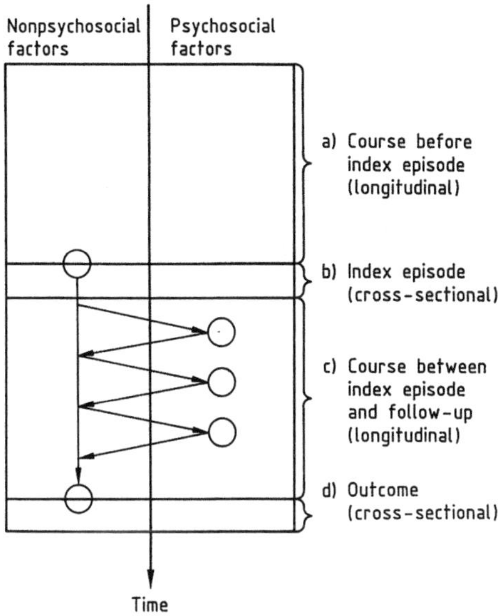

Fig. 17. Interactive developmental model

or of positive life events. Since there is a constant interaction between the individual and the environment, where the initiative may start on both sides, the term interactive is used (Fig. 17).

For example, Klerman (1974) has pointed out that depression itself exerts an influence on the nature of a person's environment. While depressed children and acutely depressed adults may elicit positive attention from the social environment, a chronic depressive adult may cause the environment to withdraw, which means that he contributes to a reduction of possible positive reinforcements in his environment. Vaughn and Leff (1976) have shown for depression that certain characteristics of the family atmosphere, called "expressed emotion," are responsible, alongside other factors, for relapses in schizophrenia. It is conceivable that the family atmosphere itself is determined by the patient and his disease and that an interactive process takes place. While the "interactive developmental model" may be the most appropriate, it is still too early to apply it in research, as Strauss et al. (1985) who have recently published a pilot study using this model, have pointed out. They have also suggested so-called longitudinal principles which can be used for describing in more detail longitudinal disease processes. They comprise nonlinearity of course; moratorium; turning points and ceilings as identifiable phases; "mountain climbing"; time decay of vulnerability (the possibility must be accounted for, that the vulnerability of the individual may change in time and that what had been a stressor at an earlier point is not a stressor at a later point or vice versa) and others. For a detailed discussion of these concepts see Strauss et al. (1985).

Study Design Problems

How depression is defined and which selection procedures are applied may clearly influence the results of a study. Few investigators have used the same diagnostic criteria. One major social factor in defining a research population is involved in the endogenous/neurotic dichotomy. The Newcastle Scale, for instance, contains among other items two "psychosocial" factors: "no adequate psychogenesis" and "premorbid personality." Practically no guidelines exist regarding how to assess "premorbid personality" and "no adequate psychogenesis," which makes these two items very unreliable. It could be shown that a change in assessing any of these items can cause a whole avalanche of patients crossing the endogenous/neurotic border of the Newcastle Scale and thus exert decisive influences on the selection of the study population (Katschnig et al. 1986a). Thus, not only if different diagnostic formulations for endogenous and neurotic populations are used, but also when one and the same definition is employed very different study populations may be obtained.

Outcomes may thus be due to the very selection of the samples. If social factors are already included in the definition of the study population in a way which does not allow to sort out to which degrees such influences played a role, a bad social outcome for neurotic depression may be simply due to the bad social situation of the patient at the index episode assessment. This is problematic in studies using ICD definitions of "neurotic depression" (e.g., Bronisch et al. 1985). Multiaxial classification systems, allowing, among others, the separate assessment of phenomenological and psychosocial factors, could help to avoid such spurious correlation between diagnostic definitions and outcome and identify the really important predictors. It is also advisable to use as many diagnostic formulations as possible, i.e., to use a polydiagnostic approach (Katschnig and Berner 1985), in order to make research results from different studies comparable with each other.

A good example for spurious correlations between diagnostic subclassification and outcome is pointed out by Coryell and Winokur (1982). In a review of existing studies on the long-term course of depressive subtypes, they commented on the discrepancies in the literature: while Kay et al. (1969) and Paykel et al. (1974) found a better prognosis for endogenous depression, Endicott and Spitzer (1979) found no difference. A closer look at the diagnostic subdivisions used in these studies reveals that in Kay et al.'s (1969) and Paykel et al.'s (1974) studies historical and personality variables had been already used for defining the diagnostic subtypes, while Endicott and Spitzer (1979) used exclusively descriptive operational criteria, namely the Research Diagnostic Criteria.

Two further diagnostic issues associated with psychosocial factors may be of decisive importance for course and outcome studies in depressive disorders. They are both concerned with the issue of chronicity. First, Akiskal et al. (1980) were able to sort out among so-called depressive personality disorders suffering from mild but chronic depression, a substantial subgroup which can be regarded as a mild form of a "real" manic-depressive illness. This group, called "subaffective dysthymia" is similar to full-blown depressive illness in many biological respects and could also be demonstrated to be responsive to antidepressive drugs. In fact, in a 4-year follow-up study, Akiskal et al. (1980) could show that not only clinical outcome but also social outcome was better in those patients with a diagnosis of "depressive personality disorders" who had responded to amitryptilin than in those who had not (and whom the authors regard as a ragbag of different types of personality disorders with psychogenic features).

A second important diagnostic issue is the concept of double depression put forward by Keller et al. (1983). By this term the authors define a clinical depressive episode which supersedes a preexisting mild but chronic form of depression. They found that such "double depression" had an especially bad prognosis, which is in line with our own findings in Vienna where the strongest predictor of subsequent chronicity was preexisting chronicity in patients suffering from a depressive episode (Katschnig and Egger-Zeidner, 1985).

Apart from such diagnostic issues, psychosocial factors play an important role in selecting patient populations into treatment facilities. This points to the need to carry out more epidemiological studies (Angst et al. 1984; Angst and Dobler-Mikola 1984a, 1984b; 1985).

It must also be mentioned that social factors are responsible for lack of cooperation in follow-up studies, i.e., for dropouts, and may thus decisively influence the characteristics of the population which one gets to cooperate in a follow-up study.The decision whether to carry out a prospective or a retrospective study must also be influenced by the consideration of psychosocial aspects. The difficulties and distortions in recall which are characteristic of all retrospective studies covering longer time periods are especially salient when psychosocial variables are studied. For instance, patients being depressed at follow-up may attribute a specific meaning to events which they would otherwise not even have remembered. On the other hand, it is frequently overlooked that repeated assessment of patients in prospective studies may in itself constitute a powerful psychosocial influence on the course of the disorder.

A deficiency of many studies is their short observation period. As Bebbington (1982) has pointed out, longer observation periods lead to worse outcome. Furthermore, it has to be considered that some events in the follow-up period may follow a specific time pattern, with, for example, higher frequencies in the beginning and lower frequencies at the end of this period.

A final methodological problem already raised by Angst (this volume), but worth mentioning again in relation to psychosocial factors, is data analysis. It is advisable to use different methods of data analysis simultaneously, since Everitt and Smith (1979) have demonstrated that traditional and log-linear methods of data analyses for the same set of data may lead to different results. It seems especially important to analyse interaction effects between psychosocial and nonpsychosocial variables. Equally, methods taking into acount the time sequence of events – such as time series analyses of life-table methods – should be applied.

Choosing Adequate Methods for Measuring Psychosocial Variables

If a realistic picture of the role of psychosocial factors in the course of depression is to be drawn, categorical psychosocial variables such as social class, marital status, or place of residence have to be supplemented by more complex and dynamic variables such as life stress, social network, social support, personality, and social adjustment. These more complex psychosocial variables are intimately connected with each other, which is rarely acknowledged in research, since they are frequently used as separate independent variables (Monroe and Steiner, 1986). Unfortunately, cheap and simple data collection methods, especially self-rating scales, still dominate psychosocial research on psychiatric disorders. When using such self-rating scales, the danger of spurious correlations between variables is increased. More elaborate and sophisticated data collection methods will have to be used than is the case at present.

The presently available data collection methods for psychopathological variables could serve as a guideline for improving data collection for psychosocial variables. Psychiatric research workers have become increasingly aware over the past two decades of the pitfalls in collecting psychopathological information, which is documented in the increasing number of rating scales and in the development of standardized clinical psychiatric interviews for collecting phenomenological information. Lengthy glossaries are supplied with these instruments, which signalizes the need for more sophisticated and cumbersome procedures in psychiatric data collection. It is true hat "quick studies," mainly in the field of psychopharmacology, still prevail, but standardized interviews become increasingly widely used and more and more research workers are, for example, trained in using the Present State Examination (Wing et al. 1984) or the Structured Clinical Interview for DSM-III (SCID; Spitzer and Williams 1984). Training and reliability studies cannot be dispensed with, if qualitatively good data is to be collected.

Such interview methods are not only imperative because of the complex nature of many psychosocial variables, but also because of their time dimension. This time dimension must be properly determined if the relationship between psychosocial and nonpsychosocial variables in the course of the disorder is to be adequately understood, since psychosocial factors may not only contribute to the development of symptoms but may also be the consequence of psychopathology. This double role of psychosocial factors both as predictor and as outcome variables deserves special methodological attention (Monroe and Steier 1986).

We will finish this section with a few remarks on especially problematic variables – personality, life events, and social support – used in course and outcome studies on depression.

Personality

It is very difficult to get a clear picture of the premorbid personality of persons who have undergone psychiatric illness episodes. If the traditional questionnaires are applied to a depressed person, retrospective assessment of personality "traits" is almost certainly contaminated with "state" variables characterizing the present depressive episode (Hirschfeld et al. 1983). It seems necessary to collect data on the premorbid personality only after the depressive episode has receded or at least improved to get as little retrospective distortion as possible, if the patient alone is questioned. In addition it seems advisable to use also other informants, such as friends or relatives (Katschnig et al. 1983). In the study by Katschnig and Egger-Zeidner (1985) the clinical judgment of the research psychiatrist about the premorbid personality of the patient, which was made during the illness episode, did not prove to be of any predictive power for the development of chronicity. However, a personality test (Freiburger Persönlichkeitsinventar, FPI; Fahrenberg et al. 1970) only applied after remission showed that "neuroticism" was significantly correlated with the development of chronicity. This finding is consistent with the results of a recent study by Hirschfeld et al. (1986). Also in this study personality was assessed after the acute symptoms had abated.

Life Events

There is a great temptation in life-events research to use simple and economic self-rating methods. It was already pointed out that life events, personality, social support, and psychopathological symptoms are closely interconnected variables and that in retrospective research designs, when all these variables are collected in a cross-sectional follow-up evaluation, there is a great danger of spurious correlations which are artefacts of the data collection method (Monroe and Steiner 1986). It seems therefore of utmost importance to use more elaborate and structured life-event methods, such as the "London Life Event and Difficulties Schedule" by Brown (1974) and to resist the temptation of using simple self-rating lists, such as the "Schedule of Recent Experience" (SRE; Holmes and Rahe 1967). A contextual measurement of life stress seems the only possible way out of the dilemma between taking too few and only the most threatening life events, on the one hand, and eliciting too many and retrospectively wrongly interpreted life events, on the other (Katschnig 1986).

Social Support

The concept of social support is still rather vague, comprising a large spectrum of ideas, starting with the simple concept that not being alone is helpful and ending with complex issues such as the quality of relationships within the social network. The more sophisticated approaches also consider possible harmfulness of social relationships and contrast this harmfulness with the possible benefit. The concept of "expressed emotion" is an example of how harmful social relatonships may be (Vaughn and Leff 1976; Brown et al. 1972). The findings of Brown and Harris (1978) also support the notion of measuring the quality of relationships, and not only the existence of a social network as such. Methods for measuring social support are not clearly delimited from methods measuring social adjustment and the terminological field in this area is still very unclear (Katschnig 1983). The size and type of a social network and the social support an individual might obtain from this network are not simply to be found in "reality" but are constantly created and modified by the individual himself (Anderson et al. 1984). Henderson (1981) has pointed out that personality factors are decisive for the kind of social network a person makes use of.

When measuring social support it is important to get also some "objective" assessment of the situation. For instance, it was shown that complaints of loneliness in old people proved to have little association with actual isolation (Roth 1983). A further methodological problem is the time dimension of social support, since there is a constant interrelationship between psychopathology, life events, and network size. Social network, measured at one point in time, may not be the same a few months later.

Conclusion

Psychosocial factors are intimately connected with depression. This at least can be concluded from the persistence with which the categorical dichotomy of depression into biological and psychosocial subtypes is upheld in psychiatric practice, research, and teaching. However, whether such a categorical subdivision does, in fact, make sense has become doubtful recently, since several research results have shown that psychosocial factors are important in a certain proportion of depressed patients regardless of which subtype they belong to. It can be seen for instance, that not only the "neurotic" but also the "endogenous" type of depression – however defined – can be precipitated by life stress (e.g., Katschnig et al. 1986a) and also that the course of affective psychosis is influenced by external social factors (e.g., Wittchen and von Zerssen 1988). Anyhow, much of the research carried out so far on the course and outcome of depression – not only research involving psychosocial variables – has furnished discrepant results, and we even seem to get further and further away from creating a coherent body of knowledge with the increasing availability of studies.

One commonly known and accepted cause for this lack of coherence in our knowledge has to be sought in the field of methodology: different study designs, different methods of defining a study population, different ways of collecting information on psychosocial factors, different lengths of follow-up periods, different or to simple outcome criteria – these and similar differences may all be responsible for the discrepancies in research results with which we have confronted the reader in the first section of this paper. In the second section some of these methodological issues have been dealt with. However, the reasons for the lack of coherence of our knowledge on the course and outcome of depressive disorders are not only due to this methodological heterogeneity, they are also rooted in a more fundamental deficiency of today's research, namely the lack of an adequate model in the framework of which longitudinal research can be carried out purposefully (Strauss et al. 1985). The still prevailing classical Kraepelinian *"natural history model,"* assuming that diseases have a specific etiology, a specific symptomatology, and a specific course pattern, seduces many research workers to collect data only at the time of the index episode and the follow-up evaluation, a strategy which necessarily leads to neglecting possible influences on the course of the disorder between these two cross sectional points in time which could account for the variance in outcome.

An alternative would be to apply the *"vulnerability-stress model"* – used so far mainly for etiolgical research – also in longitudinal studies on the course of depression. This model would accommodate stressful external events which might influence the course of a disorder during the follow-up period. If not only negative but also positive influences – positive life events or therapeutic interventions – are taken into account, this model could be extended to a *"vulnerability-external influence model."* It assumes that some biological or psychological vulnerability within the individual is activated by external stress factors (in the case of relapses) and "attenuated" by positive events or therapy (in the case of remission or absence of relapses). Clearly, the application of this model requires more intensive research efforts, since not only the two major evaluations – at the index episode and at the follow-up – have to be carried out, but also the time course in between them has to be observed. Prospective research designs using repeated evaluations after short intervals seem to be methodologically more sound than retrospective designs for collecting information about external influences during the course of a disorder; however, one has to take into consideration that repeated evaluations of a disorder during its course may themselves influence that course. In any case, whether prospectively or retrospectively collected, it seems of utmost importance in order to explain more of the variance of course and outcome of depression to take external influences operating between the index episode and the outcome evaluation into account.

Even the "vulnerability-external influence model" still seems to be too simple. External influences not only come out of the blue, but their occurrence may be influenced by the individual and the disorder itself. There is a constant interchange between individual and environment; for example, it is evident that lack of social support may be the consequence of a depressed person rejecting others and not only an independent influence towards a bad outcome. Strauss et al. (1985) have consequently proposed an *"interactive developmental model"* for studying the course and outcome of psychiatric disorders, especially schizophrenia. This is, in our opinion, the desirable direction in which also research on the course and outcome of depression has to go. However, while it may be useful to have this model in mind while doing such research, it has to be acknowledged that serious practical limitations of data collection still beset its implementation. Simple and cheap self-rating techniques may only obscure existing relationships or even produce false relationships between different variables, since in most cases they do not give the time relationship between the different variables measured. The application of an "interactive developmental model" and the use of more elaborate interview methods requiring extensive training of research workers seem to be the only promising ways of arriving at better founded conclusions on the laws governing the course of depressive disorders.

References

Agras S, Chapin N, Oliveau D (1972) The natural history of phobia: course and prognosis. Arch Gen Psychiatry 26:315–317

Akisal HS, Rosenthal TL, Haykal RF, Lemmi H, Rosenthal RH, Scott-Strauss A (1980) Characterological depression. Clinical and sleep EEG findings separating "subaffective dysthymias" from "character spectrum disorders". Arch Gen Psychiatry 37:777–783

Akisal HS, Hirschfeld RMA, Yerevanian BI (1983) The relationship of personality to affective disorders. Arch Gen Psychiatry 40:801–810

Anderson CM, Hogarty G, Bayer T, Needleman R (1984) Expressed emotion and social networks of parents of schizophrenic patients. Br J Psychiatry 144:247–255

Angst J, Dobler-Mikola A (1984a) The Zurich study. II. The continuum from normal to pathological depressive mood swings. Eur Arch Psychiatry Neurol Sci 234:21–29

Angst J, Dobler-Mikola A (1984b) The Zurich study. III. Diagnosis of depression. Eur Arch Psychiatry Neurol Sci 234:30–37

Angst J, Dobler-Mikola A (1985) The Zurich study – a prospective epidemiologcal study of depressive, neurotic and psychosomatic syndromes. IV. Recurrent and nonrecurrent brief depression. Eur Arch Psychiatry Neurol Sci 234:408–416

Angst J, Dobler-Mikola A, Binder J (1984) The Zurich study – a prospective epidemiological study of depressive, neurotic and psychosomatic syndromes. I. Problem, methodology. Eur Arch Psychiatry Neurol Sci 234:13–20

Bebbington PE (1982) The course and prognosis of affective psychoses. In: Wing JK, Wing L (eds) Handbook of psychiatry, vol 3, Psychoses of uncertain aetiology. Cambridge University Press, Cambridge, pp 120–128

Bland RC, Orn H (1983) Course and outcome in affective disorders. Can J Psychiatry 27:573–578

Bond ED, Braceland FJ (1937) Prognosis in mental disease. Am J Psychiatry 94:263–274

Bothwell S, Weissman MM (1977) Social impairments four years after an acute depressive episode. Am J Orthopsychiatry 47:231–237

Bronisch T, Wittchen H-U, Krieg C, Rupp H-U, von Zerssen D (1985) Depressive neurosis. A long-term prospective and retrospective follow-up study of former inpatients. Acta Psych Scand 71:237–248

Brown GW (1974) Meaning, measurement and stress of life events. In: Dohrenwand BS, Dohrenwand BP (eds) Stressful life events: their nature and effects. Wiley, New York, pp 217–243

Brown G, Adler WZ, Bifulco A (1988) Life events, difficulties and recovery from chronic depression. Br J Psychiatry 152:487–498

Brown G, Harris T (1978) Social origins of depression – a study of psychiatric disorders in women. Tavistock Publications, London
Brown GW, Birley JLT, Wing JK (1972) Influence of family life on the course of schizophrenic disorders: a replication. Br J Psychiatry 121:241–258
Burke L, Deykin E, Jacobson S, Haley S (1967) The depressed woman returns – a study of post-hospital adjustment. Arch Gen Psychiatry 16:548–553
Ceroni GB, Neri C, Pezzoli A (1984) Chronicity in major depression. A naturalistic prospective study. J Affective Disord 7:123–132
Clum G (1966) Intrapsychic variables and the patient's environment as factors in prognosis. Can Psychiatr Assoc J 11:131–140
Copeland JRM (1983) Psychotic and neurotic depression: discriminant function analysis and five-year outcome. Psychol Med 13:373–383
Copeland JRM (1984) Reactive and endogenous depressive illness and five-year outcome. J Affective Disord 6:153–162
Coryell W, Winokur G (1982) Course and outcome. In: E Paykel (ed) Handbook of affective disorders. Churchill Livingstone, Edinburgh, pp 93–106
Endicott J, Spitzer RL (1979) Use of the research diagnostic criteria and the "Schedule of Affective Disorders and Schizophrenia" to study affective disorders. Am J Psychiatry 136:52–56
Everitt BS, Smith AMR (1979) Interactions in contingency tables: a brief discussion of alternative definitions. Psychol Med 9:581–583
Fahrenberg J, Selg H, Hampel R (1970) Freiburger Persönlichkeitsinventar. Hogrefe, Göttingen
Goering P, Wasylenki D, Lancee W, Freeman SJJ (1983) Social support and post-hospital outcome for depressed women. Can J Psychiatry 28:612–618
Hastings DW (1958) Follow-up results in psychiatric illness. Am J Psychiatry 114:1057–1066
Henderson AS (1981) Social relationship, adversity and neurosis: an analysis of prospective observations. Br J Psychiatry 138:391–398
Henderson AS (1984) Interpreting the evidence on social support. Soc Psychiatry 19:49–52
Henderson AS, Duncan-Jones P, Byrne DG (1980) Measuring social relationships: the interview schedule for social interaction. Psychol Med 90:723–734
Hirschfeld RMA, Klerman GL, Clayton PJ, Keller MB, McDonald-Scott P, Larkin BH (1983) Assessing personality: effects of the depressive state on trait measurement. Am J Psychiatry 140:695–699
Hirschfeld RMA, Klerman GL, Andreasen NC, Clayton PJ, Keller MB (1986) Psychosocial predictors of chronicity in depressed patients. Br J Psychiatry 148:648–654
Holmes ThH, Rahe H (1967) The Social Readjustment Rating Scale. J Psychosom Res 11:213–218
Katschnig H (1983) Methods of measuring social adjustment. In: Helgason T (ed): Methodology in Evaluation of Psychiatric Treatment. Cambridge University Press, Cambridge, pp 205–218
Katschnig H (1986) Measuring life stress – a comparison of the checklist and the panel technique. In: Katschnig H (ed) Life events and psychiatric disorders – controversial issue. Cambridge University Press, Cambridge, pp 74–106
Katschnig H, Berner P (1985) The poly-diagnostic approach in psychiatric research. In: ADAMHA/WHO: Mental Disorders, Alcohol and Drug-related Problems: International Perspectives on their Diagnosis and Classification. Elsevier, Amsterdam, pp 113–120
Katschnig H, Egger-Zeidner E (1984) Depressionstyp und Depressionverlauf. In: Kryspin-Exner K, Hinterhuber H, Schubert H (eds) Langzeittherapie psychiatrischer Erkrankungen. Schattauer, Stuttgart New York, pp 7–16
Katschnig H, Egger-Zeidner E (1985) Psychosocial predictors of chronicity in depression. In: Pichot P, Berner P, Wolf R, Thau K (eds) Psychiatry: the state of the art, vol 1. Plenum, New York, pp 629–639

Katschnig H, Fuchs-Robetin G (1984) Prognose nach Suizidversuch. In: Deutsch E, Kleinberger G, Ritz R, Schuster HP (eds) Diagnose, Verlaufskontrolle und Therapie schwerer exogener Vergiftungen. Schattauer, Stuttgart, pp 243–248
Katschnig H, Angst J, Clayton PJ, Gershon ES, Hautzinger M, Helmchen H, Henderson AS, Klerman GL, Möller H-J, Paykel ES, Roth M, Weissman MM (1983) Risk factors for depression. In: Angst J (ed) The origins of depression – current concepts and approaches. Dahlem Workshop Report. Springer, Berlin Heidelberg New York
Katschnig H, Pakesch G, Egger Zeidner E (1986a) Life stress and depressive subtypes: a review of present diagnostic criteria and recent research results. In: Katschnig H (ed) Life events and psychiatric disorders – controversial issues. Cambridge University Press, Cambridge, pp 201–245
Katschnig H, Nutzinger D, Schanda H (1986b) Validating depressive subtypes. In: Hippius H, Klerman G, Matussek N (eds) New results in depression research. Springer, Berlin Heidelberg New York, pp. 36–44
Kay DWK, Garside RF, Roy JR, Beamish P (1969) "Endogenous" and "neurotic" syndromes of depression: a 5- to 7-year follow-up of 104 cases. Br J Psychiatry 115:389–399
Keller MB, Shapiro RW (1981) Major depressive disorder. Initial results from a one-year prospective naturalistic follow-up study. J Nerv Ment Dis 169:761–768
Keller MB, Lavori PW, Endicott J, Coryell W, Klerman GL (1983) "Double depression" – a two year follow-up. Am J Psychiatr 140:689–694
Kerr TA, Roth M, Schapira K, Gurney C (1972) The assessment and prediction of outcome in affective disorders. Br J Psychiatry 121:167–174
Klerman GL (1974) Depression and adaptation. In: Friedman RJ, Katz MM (eds) The psychology of depression: contemporary theory and research. Wiley, New York, pp 127–156
Klerman GL (1980) Long-term outcome of neurotic depressions. In: Sells SB, Crandall R, Roff M, Strauss JS, Pollin W (eds) Human functioning in longitudinal perspective. Williams and Wilkins, Baltimore London, pp 58–73
Kraepelin E (1909) Psychiatrie, 8th edn. Barth, Leipzig
Merikangas KR, Bromet EJ, Spiker DG (1983) Assortative mating, social adjustment and course of illness in primary affective disorder. Arch Gen Psychiatry 40:795–800
Monroe SM, Steiner S (1986) Social support and psychopathology: interrelation with preexisting disorders, stress and personality. J Abn Psych 95:29–39
Monroe SM, Thase ME, Hersen M, Himmelhoch JM, Bellack AS (1985) Life events and the endogenous-nonendogenous distinction in the treatment and posttreatment course of depression. Comp Psychiatry 26:175–186
Paykel ES, Klerman GL, Prusoff BA (1974) Prognosis of depression and the endogenous-neurotic distinction. Psychol Med 4:57–64
Perris H (1984) Life events and depression. Part 2. Results in diagnostic subgroups, and in relation to the recurrence of depression. J Affective Disord 7:25–36
Prusoff BA, Weissman MM, Klerman GL, Rounsaville BJ (1980) Research diagnostic criteria subtypes of depression. Their role as predictors of differential response to psychotherapy and drug treatment. Arch Gen Psychiatry 37:796–801
Rennie TAC (1942) Prognosis in manic-depressive psychoses. Am J Psychiatry 98:801–814
Roth M (1983) Depression and affective disorder in later life. In: Angst J (ed) The origins of depression: Current concepts and approaches. Dahlem Konferenzen, Springer, Berlin Heidelberg New York Tokyo, pp 39–75
Schapira K, Roth M, Kerr TA, Gurney C (1972) The prognosis of affective disorders: the differentiation of anxiety states from depressive illnesses. Br J Psychiatry 121:175–181
Shobe FO, Brion P (1971) Long-term prognosis in manic-depressive illness: a follow-up investigation of 111 patients. Arch Gen Psychiatry 24:334–337
Spitzer RL, Williams JB (1984) Structured Clinical Interview for DSM-III. Biometric Research Department, New York

Strauss JS, Hafez H, Lieberman P, Harding CM (1985) The course of psychiatric disorder, III. Longitudinal principles. Am J Psychiatry 142:289–296
Strömgren E (1974) Psychogenetic psychoses. In: Themes and variation in European psychiatry. Hirsch S, Shephard M (eds) Wright, Bristol, pp 79–117
Surtees PG (1980) Social support, residual adversity and depressive outcome. Soc Psychiatry 15:71–80
Swift HM (1907–1908) The prognosis of recurrent insanity of the manic-depressive type. Am J Insanity 64:311–326
Tennant C, Bebbington P, Hurry J (1981 a) The short-term outcome of neurotic disorders in the community: the relation of remission to clinical factors and to "neutralizing" life events. Br J Psychiatry 139:213–220
Tennant C, Hurry J, Bebbington P (1981 b) The short-term outcome of neurotic disorders in the community – demographic and clinical predictors of remission. Aust NZ J Psychiatry 15:111–116
Vaughn CE, Leff JP (1976) The influence of family life and social factors on the course of psychiatric illness. Br J Psychiatry 129:125–137
Weissman MM, Klerman GL, Paykel ES, Prusoff BA, Hanson B (1974) Treatment effects on the social adjustment of depressed patients. Arch Gen Psychiatry 30:771–778
Weissman MM, Prusoff BA, Klerman GL (1978) Personality and the prediction of long-term outcome of depression. Am J Psychiatry 135:797–800
Wimmer A (1916) Psykogene Sindssygdromsformer (Psychogene Geisteskrankheitsformen) In: St Hans Hospital 1816–1916. Jubiläumsschrift, Copenhagen, pp 85–216
Wing JK, Cooper JE, Sartorius N (1974) The measurement and classification of psychiatric symptoms. Cambridge University Press, London.
Wittchen H-U, von Zerssen D (1988) Verläufe behandelter und unbehandelter affektiver Störungen. Springer, Berlin Heidelberg New York

Comments

V. Lehtinen

There is still considerable controversy as to the definition, diagnostics, epidemiology, clinical course, and treatment of depression. The place of depression in nosological classification systems has continued to be problematic and this problem should be explicitly recognized and discussed. In fact, when we here talk about depressive disorders and the psychological and social factors affecting their clinical course and outcome, we cannot actually be sure that what we mean by "depressive disorders" is the same in each case. Such a consensus, however, would be of the most fundamental importance.

I consider it particularly important that Professor Katschnig stressed in his paper factors related to study design and methodology. I myself must agree with most of the views he has put forth. Just as I have emphasized the problematic nature of the definition of the concept of depression (and the recognition of such problems), the defintion and operationalization problems related to many psychosocial factors must naturally also be made explicit. As Katschnig points out, the same psychosocial factors can act both as the cause of the disorder and as its consequences. In practice, there are probably often complex interactional processes, and it is, to say the least, not a simple matter to keep these under control using ordinary research methods and data analyzing techniques. We can probably approach the problem somewhat more closely through systems-theory and cybernetic models, but, at the same time, the methodological problems become even more accentuated.

I think that the question concerning the natural course of depression and spontaneous recovery is a theoretically interesting one, and fundamental in terms of the topic of our workshop. Although Professor Katschnig brings up with good reason the problems related to the "natural history paradigm," I feel that we should not completely give up the effort to study this topic, too. Of course it is clear that every individual who suffers from depression has his own historical uniqueness. His depression and its course are linked with a highly individual and complex combination of biological, psychological, and social factors. Despite this, however, we may find grounds that justify our considering depression in a certain sense also to be an independent phenomenon, at least if the cultural environment and point in time are the same.

Department of Psychiatry, University Central Hospital of Turku, SF-20520 Turku

Depressive Illness: Prediction of Course and Outcome
Edited by T. Helgason and R. J. Daly

Finally, let me give my own list of the areas in which our knowledge is too scanty or inconsistent and which I consider fundamental in terms of our own topic. I will list these areas without further comment:

1. The natural course of depression (e.g., the duration of the illness episodes, subclinical manifestations, the tendency towards fluctuation)
2. The incidence of depression and associated psychological factors
3. The factors related to recovery from depression (treatment, psychosocial factors)
4. Depression and personal loss (both concrete and symbolic)
5. The epidemiology of masked depression and forms taken by it (e.g., indirect, self-destructive behavior)

Biological Aspects of Course and Outcome in Depressive Illness: Needed Areas of Research

N. Matussek

Introduction

On the basis of the results obtained in clinical biologic-psychiatric depression research, prediction of course and outcome in a depressive illness is still not possible. Nevertheless, in the past decade a number of different groups have worked out quite a few interesting outlines for elucidating the questions treated in this symposium and which must be further pursued.

Before, however, discussing some special neurobiologic results which could be important with regard to our topic, I would like to mention a fundamental problem which should be principally considered in biologic-psychiatric depression research in order to obtain concomitant results. That is to say that the patients who are included in often longitudinal, highly sophisticated and expensive studies, should be described more precisely than has usually been done so far. We know that a depressive syndrome with its diverse symptomatology may be due to different causes, and we have to assume that both different symptomatology and different genesis produce different somatic and neurobiologic changes in the body. Above all – and already Kraepelin stressed this again and again at the turn of this century – it is particularly important to consider accurately the course of a psychiatric disorder for the purpose of coming to a most clear classification. In my opinion, in all classification systems at hand (ICD, DSM III, RCD, etc.) the course criteria of a depressive syndrome are not well enough considered. Subdividing such syndromes into endogenous, neurotic, or reactive depressions, and major or minor depressive episodes is predominantly done according to the symptomatology and less in consideration of the course of the disorder, which is not sufficient for many biologic-psychiatric research projects. Therefore, at the Dahlem Conferences 1983 (Angst 1983), our working group set up some „Recommendations for Reporting Clinical Studies of Functional Indices of Biologic Disturbances" which in the meantime have been published by Kupfer and Rush (1983). It would be desirable if these „Recommendations" were more and more applied worldwide. Thus, depressive patients included in biologic-psychiatric research projects could be more accurately defined independently of the rough classificati-

Nervenklinik der Universität München, Psychiatrische Klinik und Poliklinik, Nußbaumstr. 7, D-8000 München 2

Depressive Illness: Prediction of Course and Outcome
Edited by T. Helgason and R. J. Daly

on and more homogenous subgroups of affective disorders could be obtained which would then be characterized biologically.

Cerebrospinal Fluid 5-Hydroxyindolacetic Acid (CSF 5-HIAA)

Following the serotonin-deficit hypothesis (Coppen 1967; Lapin and Oxenkrug 1969; van Praag 1979), a great number of autopsy and CSF studies showed at least some depressive patients to have a reduced 5-HIAA concentration in certain brain areas or in the CSF (review; Matussek 1980). Since affective disorders were found to be more frequent in relatives of patients with low CSF 5-HIAA than in the families of patients with normal 5-HIAA values, van Praag and de Haan (1979) concluded that a low 5-HIAA concentration in CSF might be a factor of vulnerability to depression. The studies of Sedvall et al. (1980) suggest the same interpretation, since nondepressive probands with a family history of affective disorders were found to have lower lumbal CSF 5-HIAA values than probands without family history of affective disorders. Besides, we have to consider that reduced lumbal CSF 5-HIAA values were equally found in alcoholism (Ballenger et al. 1979) as well as in obsessive-compulsive disorders (Thorén et al. 1980), i.e., in diseases that are connected to the affective disorders.

Furthermore, in most of the investigations, a higher risk for suicide attempts was found in depressive patients with reduced CSF 5-HIAA concentrations (review; Åsberg et al. 1985). I agree with the authors in interpreting this finding as evidence of a negative correlation between autoaggression and serotonin (5-HT) turnover. In other studies sociopaths with high aggression scores, but without depression, were found to have low lumbar CSF 5-HIAA values (Brown et al. 1982a, 1982b). Very brutal murderers equally belong to the group having low CSF 5-HIAA values (Åsberg et al. 1985). Furthermore, a number of animal experimental investigations suggest relations between 5-HT metabolism and aggression. A blockade of the 5-HT synthesis with PCPA, a serotonin antagonist, particularly in combination with DOPA (Lyche et al. 1969; Benkert et al. 1973), as well as isolation (Garattini et al. 1967), induce a marked increase of the fighting behavior. Neurophysiologic studies, too, show the firing rate of dorsal raphe neurons to be decreased in offensive animals (tree shrew), whereas it is increased in defensive animals (Walletschek and Raab 1982). It is quite clear today, that there is a strong correlation between 5-HT turnover in the brain and aggression. On the other hand, we have to consider that isolated or PCPA-treated animals cannot serve as depression models, but that the contrary may be the case. PCPA-treated animals show motor (Benkert et al. 1973) and sexual (Tagliamonte et al. 1969) hyperactivity. Thus, for the autoaggression of depressive patients further neurobiologic disturbances must be postulated in addition to the functional 5-HT deficit to explain a depressive-suicidal syndrome. Whether adrenoceptors could be involved will be discussed in the next section. According to the data obtained so far, which can only briefly be referred to, persons with low lumbar CSF 5-HIAA values seem to represent an important risk group to which greater attention has to be paid in the future. To my knowledge there are to date no studies proving whether a treatment combination of tryptophan plus MAO inhibitor or 5-hydroxytryptophan plus decarboxylase inhibitor, which have both been successfully applied to the treatment of depression, would positively influence a suicidal syndrome or aggressive sociopathic behavior.

Adrenoceptors

On the basis of results available to date the original noradrenaline (NA) hypothesis of depression introduced by Everett and Toman (1959) which was extended by Schildkraut (1965), Bunney and Davis (1965), and Matussek (1966) can no longer be maintained (review, Matussek 1980). Neuroendocrine investigations in depressive patients suggest that there is rather a reduced α-adrenoceptor sensitivity than a NA deficit involved at least in endogenous depression. The growth hormone (GH) response to clonidine, an α-2-adrenoceptor agonist, was shown to be significantly reduced in endogenous as compared with neurotic-reactive depressive patients and controls (Matussek et al. 1980). This finding has since been confirmed by other study groups (Checkley et al. 1981; Charney et al. 1982a; Siever et al. 1982a; Boyer et al. 1983; Ansseau et al. 1984; Checkley et al. 1984). The findings of Laakmann et al. (1980) who used desmethylimipramine (DMI) to stimulate GH, and which have been confirmed in 1982 by Sawa et al., point in the same direction. The DMI-induced GH stimulation can be blocked with phentolamine, a postsynaptic α-1- and α-2-adrenoceptor antagonist, whereas prazosin, a selective α-1-adrenergic antagonist, exerts no influence on the DMI-induced GH stimulation (Laakmann et al. 1986a).

Checkley and Crammer (1977) and Checkley (1979) interpreted their results concerning the methylamphetamine effect on cortisol secretion in endogenous as compared with reactive depressive patients and controls also as a reduced α-adrenoceptor sensitivity. The ACTH cortisol secretion does seem to be stimulated by α-1- and not by α-2-adrenoceptors (Laakmann et al. 1986b). However, all findings obtained with the clonidine GH stimulation test reveal that a reduced α-2-adrenoceptor sensitivity is not the only or specific factor responsible for the occurrence of a depressive phase. Postmenopausal females (Matussek et al. 1980; Siever et al. 1982a, b), women in the menstruation period, as well as probands who regularly consume alcohol likewise have a blunted GH response to clonidine, without being depressive (Matussek et al. 1984). Thus, further, so far unknown factors must also be involved in provoking a depressive phase. Due to the reciprocal balance of α- and β-adrenoceptors (Kunos 1980; U'Prichard 1984), one might suppose that the so-called „β-down-regulation“ after repeated application of antidepressant drugs or ECT (Sulser 1982) could be linked with an up-regulation of α-adrenoceptors. The reciprocal modulation of α- and β-adrenergic receptors has been previously demonstrated, particularly with regard to GH secretion. β-Adrenergic receptor blockers increase, whereas β-agonists decrease GH stimulation (Brown et al. 1979). Laakmann et al. (1986 a) showed the same finding with DMI. Since the α-adrenoceptor sensitivity is influenced by the endorphine system (Eriksson et al. 1981) and the „β-down-regulation" affected both by serotonergic (Brunello et al. 1982; Janowsky et al. 1982) and GABA-ergic (Enna et al. 1984) neuronal systems, as well as by adrenocortical and sexual hormones (Sulser 1982), intensive efforts are necessary for elucidating the reciprocal actions of the different neuronal and hormone systems in regulating the different adrenoceptors. Whether this will help to detect the mechanism provoking an endogenous depressive phase or to understand the therapeutic action of antidepressant drugs must be assessed by future studies.

Based on our first results obtained with the clonidine GH stimulation test (Matussek et al. 1980), we thought the blunted GH response to clonidine to be possibly a marker of vulnerability for endogenous depression. Since it did not alter under antidepressant treatment, Charney et al. (1982 b) and Corn et al. (1984 a, b) supposed the blunted GH response to clonidine to be a trait marker for depression. In eight of nine endogenous depressive patients in the free interval and without medication for at least 6 weeks, we found the GH response to clonidine still blunted (Höhe et al. 1986). For all these reasons we, too, would regard the blunted GH response to clonidine, i.e., the reduced α-2-adrenoceptor sensitivity, possibly as a trait marker for endogenous depression. Also other authors did not find the GH response to clonidine to be altered under antidepressant treatment (Siever et al. 1982 b; Charney et al. 1982 b; Corn et al. 1984 a), whereas Glass et al. (1982), as well as our group (Matussek et al. 1985) in six of eight endogenous depressive patients found an increased GH response in the course of antidepressant treatment. Further studies, which have to consider the menstruation cycle, alcohol, and medication anamnesis, are necessary to check whether the GH response to clonidine changes under antidepressant treatment. If, as mentioned above, there is a reciprocal balance between α- and β-adrenoceptors and a "β-down-regulation" under antidepressant drugs in man as well, one should expect an increase of the α-2-mediated GH response to clonidine, which should decrease again in the course of treatment, as has been found by Glass et al. (1982) in patients and by Corn et al. (1984 b) in healthy probands. Actually, we do to date not yet exactly understand the molecular-biologic mechanisms responsible for the regulation between α- and β-adrenoceptors. Elucidation of these mechanisms seems of great importance for biologic-psychiatric depression research.

Tyramine Challenge Test

Some time ago already Merton Sandler's group found that, following oral tyramine load, depressive patients showed a significant decrease in urinary output of sulfate conjugated tyramine as compared to controls (Sandler et al. 1975; Bonham Carter et al. 1978). Likewise, in a group of normal pregnant women after an oral tyramine load, women with a signficantly higher lifetime incidence of depression had a significantly lower output of urinary tyramine (Bonham Carter et al. 1980). The authors suggested this test to be a trait marker for depression (Sandler et al. 1983). These findings have been confirmed and extended since then. Of 101 depressed outpatients, unipolar and bipolar patients with DSM-III criteria for melancholia produced a significant, abnormally low tyramine sulfate excretion as compared to atypical and mood-reactive depressions and controls (Harrison et al. 1984). In this study, too, 12 patients in remission after recovery from episodes of melancholia and free of psychotropic medication showed an abnormally low tyramine sulfate excretion. The authors suggest the tyramine challenge test to be a marker for melancholia. Recent investigations by Sandler's group (Hale et al. 1985) show that in this test endogenous discriminate from nonendogenous depressive patients. "The degree of conjugation deficiency appears to be independent of clinical severity of depression." To date the cause of this biochemical lesion could not be clarified. Further studies with regard to course and outcome of affective disorders and to the responsible biochemical mechanism are necessary.

Peptides and Adrenaline in CSF

Discovery of a great number of neuropeptides in the past 15 years raised hopes also in biologic-psychiatric depression research. Many a high expectation has not been fulfilled to date in this field. Interesting, but not always concomitant results in the peptide field in connection with affective disorders have, e.g., been obtained with the TRH/TSH test as agent for the diagnosis and for the prediction of the course (review, Prange and Loosen 1984). Since we do not yet completely know the neurobiologic mechanisms of a great many of these neuromodulators, we have to await development of basic research in this field and to see whether new aspects will be outlined which could be relevant for depression research.

In this connection I would, however, like to mention one interesting finding in the field of peptides. O. Rafaelsen's group measured in CSF of patients with endogenous depression, nonendogenous depression, mania, schizophrenia, and in neurological controls: vasoactive intestinal polypeptide (VIP), cholecystokinin (CCK), gastrin, vasopressin, and thyreotropin releasing hormone (TRH; Gjerris et al. 1981 a, b). Only in the group of nonendogenous depressive patients they found a significantly lower CSF-VIP amount with no increase or normalization following clinical recovery. The authors ask whether low CSF-VIP could be a marker for this type of depression. There is to date no neurobiological explanation for the VIP deficit. There was no difference found in all other peptides measured in CSF.

CSF noradrenaline (NA) and adrenaline (A) were also determined in the course of the above investigations. NA values did not differ between endogenous and nonendogenous depressions and controls, while the A values of both groups of depressive patients during the depressive phase were significantly reduced as compared to controls – after recovery they increased by 200%–300%. It seems necessary that other groups extend these results, which have been found in a small number of patients only in order to assess whether by means of these tests state or trait markers for depression can be discriminated.

Conclusion

For many years a great number of research groups worldwide have made many efforts to elucidate the neurobiological functions in affective disorders. So far no unequivocal, generally accepted, and reproducible results have been obtained. We do not yet know the neurobiologic changes of brain functions during an endogenous, neurotic, or reactive depression responsible for the symptomatology. Many studies suggest disturbances in the brain 5-HT or NA metabolism, which are all not specific for depression. The same must be stated regarding the results found in the hypothalamus-pituitary adrenal cortex and -thyroid system, which have often been discussed but not have been included here. Likewise, the results concerning the imipramine binding in platelets of depressive patients (Rehavi et al. 1984) could not always be confirmed, although methodological determination problems might be responsible for the divergent results.

In my opinion it is particularly important for future studies that specific investigations should be carried out in depressive patients with different etiology, after recovery from the depressive phase, who have to be drug-free, in order to assess in a larger number of patients whether CSF 5-HIAA or VIP, GH response to clonidine or DMI, H^3-imipraminebinding in platelets, or the tyramine challenge might be adequate tests for detecting trait or state markers for certain forms of depression. It would be most desirable that every patient should be characterized by as many biologic parameters as possible, that the course of the disease should be documented longitudinally, and that the family or even better monozygotic twins, especially if they are discordant in respect of depression, should be included. Since in endogenous depressions today an early prophylactic treatment is carried through, such interval studies would already have to be performed after the second depressive phase. Due to the great importance of the corticosteroids and the thyroid system, these hormones have to be considered as well in order to recognize the neurobiologic mechanisms inducing a depressive phase. Since not all determination methods are available in all laboratories and since patients who are psychopathologically and in their course of illness well characterized, and who are willing to cooperate, are not very frequent, cooperation between different centers would be necessary to come to a higher number of patients included in such studies. We have to wait and see whether it will be possible, with our insufficient knowledge of the manifold interactions in the central nervous system and with the methods available, to clarify the neurobiologic dysfunctions connected with the different depressive syndromes.

References

Angst J (1983) The origins of depression: current concepts and approaches (Dahlem Konferenzen). Life Sciences Research Report 26. Springer, Berlin Heidelberg New York Tokyo

Ansseau M, Scheyvaerts M, Doumont A, Poirrier R, Legros JJ, Franck G (1984) Concurrent use of REM latency, dexamethasone suppression, clonidine, and apomorphine tests as biological markers of endogenous depression: a pilot study. Psychiatry Res 12:261–272

Åsberg M, Martensson B, Wägner A (1985) Biochemical markers of serotonin functions in depression and suicidal behaviour. In: Hippius H, Klerman G, Matussek N (eds) New results in depression research. Springer, Berlin Heidelberg New York Tokyo

Ballenger JC, Goodwin FK, Major LF, Brown GC (1979) Alcohol and central serotonin metabolism in man. Arch Gen Psychiatry 36:224–227

Benkert O, Renz A, Matussek N (1973) Dopamine, noradrenaline, 5-hydroxytryptamine in relation to motor activity, fighting and mounting behaviour. II. L-Dopa and DL-threo-dihydroxyphenyl-alanine. Neuropharmacology 12:187–193

Bonham Carter SM, Sandler M, Goodwin BL, Sepping P, Bridges PK (1978) Decreased urinary output of tyramine and its metabolites in depression. Br J Psychiatry 132:125–132

Bonham Carter SM, Revely MA, Sandler M, Dewhurst J, Little BC, Hayworth J, Priest RG (1980) Decreased urinary output of conjugated tyramine is associated with lifetime vulnerability of depressive illness. Psychiatry Res 3:13–31

Boyer P, Schaub C, Guelfi JD, Nassiet J, Pichot P (1983) Growth hormone response to hypothalamic-α-receptor stimulation in depressive states. VII. World congress of Psychiatry, Vienna

Brown GL, Friend WC, Chambers JW (1979) Neuropharmacology of hypothalamic-pituitary regulation. In: Tolis G, Labrie F, Martin JB, Naftolin F (eds) Clinical neuroendocrinology. A pathophysiological approach. Raven Press, New York, pp 47–81

Brown GL, Goodwin FK, Bunney WE (1982a) Human aggression and suicide: their relationship to neuropsychiatric diagnoses and serotonin metabolism. In: Ho BT et al. (eds) Serotonin in biological psychiatry. Raven Press, New York, pp 287–307

Brown GL, Ebert MH, Goyer PF, Jimerson DC, Klein WJ, Bunney WE, Goodwin FK (1982b) Aggression, suicide, and serotonin: relationships to CSF amine metabolites. Am J Psychiatry 139:741–746

Brunello N, Barbaccia ML, Chuang DM, Costa E (1982) Downregulation of β-adrenergic receptors following repeated injections of desmethylimipramine: permissive role of serotonergic axons. Neuropharmacology 21:1145–1149

Bunney WE, Davis JM (1985) Norepinephrine in depressive reactions. Arch Gen Psychiatry 13:483

Charney DS, Heninger GR, Sternberg DE, Hafstad KM, Ginnings S, Landis DH (1982a) Adrenergic receptor sensitivity in depression: effects of clonidine in depressed patients and healthy subjects. Arch Gen Psychiatry 39:290–294

Charney DS, Heninger GR, Sternberg DE (1982b) Failure of chronic antidepressant treatment to alter growth hormone response to clonidine. Psychiatry Res 7:135–138

Charney DS, Heninger GR, Sternberg DE (1984) The effect of mianserin on alpha-2 adrenergic receptor function in depressed patients. Br J Psychiatry 144:407–416

Checkley SA (1979) Corticosteroid and growth hormone responses to methylamphetamine in depressive illness. Psychol Med 9:107–115

Checkley SA, Crammer JL (1977) Hormone responses to methylamphetamine in depression: a new approach to the noradrenaline depletion hypothesis. Br J Psychiatry 131:582–586
Checkley SA, Slade AP, Shur E (1981) Growth hormone and other responses to clonidine in patients with endogenous depression. Br J Psychiatry 138:51–55
Chekley SA, Glass IB, Thompson C, Corn T, Robinson P (1984) The GH response to clonidine in endogenous as compared with reactive depression. Psychol Med 14:773–777
Coppen A (1967) The biochemistry of affective disorders. Br J Psychiatry 113:1237–1264
Corn TH, Honig A, Thompson C, Bridges PK, Bartlett JR, Checkley SA (1984a) A neuroendocrine study of stereotactic subcaudate tractotomy. Br J Psychiatry 144:417–420
Corn TH, Thompson C, Checkley SA (1984b) Effects of desipramine treatment upon central adrenoreceptor function in normal subjects. Br J Psychiatry 145:139–145
Enna SJ, Karbon EW, Duman RS (1984) GABA-B-agonists and imipramine-induced modifications in rat brain, beta-adrenergic receptor binding and function. Symposium International "GABA et les Maladies Affectives: Approche Expérimentale et Clinique," Paris, 1984
Eriksson E, Eden S, Modigh K (1981) Importance of norepinephrine alpha-2-receptor activation for morphine-induced rat growth hormone secretion. Neuroendocrinology 33:91–96
Everett GM, Toman JEP (1959) Mode of action of Rauwolfia alkaloids and motor activity. In: Masserman JH (ed) Biological Psychiatry, vol 1. Grune and Stratton, New York
Garattini S, Giacolone E, Valzelli L (1967) Isolation, aggressiveness and brain 5-hydroxytryptamine turnover. J Pharm Pharmacol 19:338–339
Gjerris A, Fahrenkrug J, Bojholm S, Rafaelsen OJ (1981a) Vasoactive intestinal polypeptide (VIP) in cerebrospinal fluid in psychiatric disorders. In: Perris C, Struwe G, Jansson B (eds) Biological psychiatry. Elsevier/Biochemical, Amsterdam, pp 359–362
Gjerris A, Jensen E, Christensen NJ, Rafaelsen O (1981b) Adrenaline and noradrenaline in psychiatric disorders. In: Perris C, Struwe G, Jansson B (eds) Biological psychiatry. Elsevier/North-Holland and Biomedical, Amsterdam, pp 565–568
Glass IB, Checkley SA, Shur E, Dawling S (1982) The effect of desipramine upon central adrenergic function in depressed patients. Br J Psychiatry 141:372–376
Hale AS, Walker PL, Bridges PK, Sandler M (1986) Tyramine conjugation deficit as a trait-marker for endogeneous depressive illness. J Psychiatr Res 20:251–261
Harrison WM, Cooper TB, Stewart JW, Quitkin FM, McGrath PJ, Leibowitz MR, Rabkin JR, Markowitz JS, Klein DF (1984) The tyramine challenge test as a marker for melancholia. Arch Gen Psychiatry 41: 681–685
Höhe M, Valido G, Matussek N (1986) Growth hormone response to clonidine in endogenous depressive patients: evidence for a trait marker in depression. In: Shagass C, Iosiassen EC, Bridger WH, Weiss KJ, Stoff D, Simpson GM (eds) Biological psychiatry 1985. Proc. IVth world congress of biological psychiatry. Elsevier, New York, pp 862–864 (Developments in psychiatry, vol 7)
Janowsky A, Okaka F, Manier DH, Applegate CD, Sulser F (1982) Role of serotonergic input in the regulation of the β-adrenergic receptor-coupled adenylate cyclase system. Science 218:900–901
Kunos G (1980) Reciprocal changes in α- and β-adrenoreceptor reactivity – myth or reality? Trends Pharmacol Sci 7:282–284
Kupfer DJ, Rush AJ (1983) Recommendations for depression publications. Psychiatry Res 8:238–240
Laakmann G (1980) Beeinflussung der Hypophysenvorderlappen-Hormonsekreation durch Antidepressiva bei gesunden Probanden, neurotisch und endogen depressiven Patienten. Nervenarzt 51:725–732
Laakmann G, Wittmann M, Schoen HW, Zygan K, Weiss A, Meissner R, Mueller OA, Stalla GK (1986a) Effects of receptor blockers (methysergide, propranolol, phentolamine, yohimbine, and prazosin) on the desimipramine-induced pituitary hormone stimulations in humans. Part III: PHA axis. Psychoneuroendocrinology 11:475–489

Laakmann G, Zygan K, Schoen HW, Weiss A, Wittmann M, Meissner R, Blaschke D (1986b) Effects of receptor blockers (methysergide, propranolol, phentolamine, yohimbine, and prazosin) on the desimipramine-induced pituitary hormone stimulation in humans. Part I: Growth hormone. Psychoneuroendocrinology 11:447–461
Lapin IP, Oxenkrug GF (1969) Intensification of the central serotonergic processes as a possible determinant of the thymoleptic effect. Lancet I:132
Lycke E, Modigh K, Roos B-E (1969) Aggression in mice associated with changes in the monoamine metabolism of the brain. Experientia 25:951–953
Matussek N (1966) Neurobiologie und Depression. Med Wochenschr 20:109
Matussek N (1980) Stoffwechselpathologie der Zyklothymie und Schizophrenie. In: Kisker KP, Meyer JE, Müller C, Strömgren E (eds) Psychiatrie der Gegenwart, vol I/2. Springer, Berlin Heidelberg New York, pp 65–113
Matussek N, Ackenheil M, Hippius H, Müller F, Schröder H-Th, Schultes H, Wasilewski B (1980) Effect of clonidine on growth hormone release in psychiatric patients and controls. Psychiatry Res 2:25–36
Matussek N, Ackenheil M, Herz M (1984) The dependence of the clonidine growth hormone test on alcohol drinking habits and the menstrual cycle. Psychoneuroendocrinology 9:173–177
Matussek N, Ackenheil M, Höhe M, Müller-Spahn F (1986) Clonidine growth-hormone stimulation test in depressive patients before and after treatment: results and methodological considerations. In: Shagass C, Tosiassen RC, Bridger WH, Weiss KJ, Stoff D, Simpson GM (eds) Biological psychiatry 1985. Proc. IVth world congress of biological psychiatry. Elsevier, New York, pp 788–790 (Developments in psychiatry, vol 7)
van Praag HM (1969) Monoamines and depression. Pharmakopsychiatrie 2:151–160
van Praag HM, de Haan S (1979) Central serotonin metabolism and the frequency of depression. Psychiatry Res 1:219–224
Prange AJ, Loosen PT (1984) Peptides in depression. In: Usdin E, Åsberg M, Bertilsson L, Sjöqvist F (eds) Frontiers in biochemical and pharmacological research in depression, vol 39. Raven Press, New York, pp 127–145
Rehavi M, Skolnick P, Paul SM (1984) High-binding sites for tricyclic antidepressants in brain and platelets. In: Marangos PJ, Campell IC, Cohen RM (eds) Brain receptor methodologies, part B. Academic Press, London, pp 279–295
Sandler M, Bonham Carter SM, Cuthbert MF, Pare CMB (1975) Is there an increase in monoamine oxidase activity in depressive illness? Lancet I:1045–1049
Sandler M, Bonham Carter SM, Walker PL (1983) Tyramine conjugation deficit as a trait-marker in depression. Psychopharmacol Bull 19:501–502
Sawa Y, Odo S, Nakasawa T (1982) Growth hormone secretion by tricyclic and non-tricyclic antidepressants in healthy volunteers and depressives. In: Kanger SZ, Takahashi R, Segawa T, Briley M (eds) New vistas in depression. Pergamon, New York, pp 309–315
Schildkraut JJ (1965) The catecholamine hypothesis of affective disorders: a review of supporting evidence. Am J Psychiatry 122:509
Sedvall G, Fyrö B, Gullberg B, Nybäck H, Wiesel F-A, Wode-Helgodt B (1980) Relationships in healthy volunteers between concentrations of monoamine metabolites in cerebrospinal fluid and family history of psychiatric morbidity. Br J Psychiatry 136:366–374
Siever LS, Uhde TW, Silberman EK, Jimerson DC, Aloi JA, Post RM, Murphy DL (1982a) The growth hormone response to clonidine as a probe of noradrenergic receptor responsiveness in affective disorder patients and controls. Psychiatry Res 6:171–183
Siever LS, Uhde TW, Insel TR, Roy BF, Murphy DL (1982b) Growth hormone response to clonidine unchanged by chronic chlorgyline treatment. Psychiatry Res 7:139–144
Sulser F (1982) Antidepressant drug research: its impact on neurobiology and psychobiology. In: Costa E, Racagni G (eds) Typical and atypical antidepressants: molecular mechanisms. Raven Press, New York, pp 1–20

Tagliamonte A, Tagliamonte P, Gessa GL, Brodie BB (1969) Compulsive sexual activity induced by p-chorophenylalanine in normal and pinealectomized male rats. Science 166:1433–1435

Thorén P, Åsberg M, Bertilson L, Mellström B, Sjöqvist F, Träskman L (1980) Chlorimipramine treatment of obsessive-compulsive disorder. Part I. Biochemical aspects. Arch Gen Psychiatry 37:1289–1295

U'Prichard DC (1984) Biochemical characteristics and regulation of brain α-2-adrenoreceptors. In: Salama AI (ed) Presynaptic modulation of postsynaptic receptors in mental diseases. Ann NY Acad Sci 430:55–75

Walletschek H, Raab A (1982) Spontaneous activity of dorsal raphe neurons during defensive and offensive encounters in the tree-shrew. Psychol Behav 28:697–705

Biological Aspects of Course and Outcome in Depressive Illness: Needed Areas of Research. N. Matussek

Comments

B. E. Leonard

The ancients postulated that melancholia was caused by an excess of "black bile" and despite the failure of investigators to identify the nature of this substance in the intervening 2000 years, the search for its identity continues. Professor Matussek, in his presentation, summarizes the evidence in favour of the "black bile" hypothesis but, in my view, correctly concludes that more thorough multidisciplinary and multicentred studies, to which a rigid clinical protocol is applied, must be undertaken before any reliable conclusions may be drawn.

Despite the plethora of incomplete and poorly controlled studies which have clouded the literature in recent years, the hypothesis that an abnormality(ies) in central neurotransmitter function underlies the affective disorders still seems credible. The main problem occurs when one tries to identify those biochemical changes which may be causally related to depressive illness and which may serve to predict response to treatment. Despite the attempts that have been made to relate changes in the CSF concentrations of monoamine metabolites to the severity of the disease (Schildkraut et al. 1978; Van Praag and de Hahn 1979), the contribution of amine metabolites from the spinal cord and the variation in CSF concentrations due to exercise and stress make it difficult to draw any firm conclusions regarding the reliability of such findings to the aetiology of depression (see review by Leonard 1982). Despite the promising report of Sacchetti et al. (1979) that it was possible to divide depressed patients into those with a noradrenaline-deficient from those with a serotonin-deficient disease based on a analysis of the metabolite concentration of the CSF, detailed and critical studies by Montgomery (1982) and Veith et al. (1983) have failed to support this hypothesis. While it may be argued that studies demonstrating a significant reduction in CSF-5 hydroxyindoleacetic acid (5-HIAA) levels are predictive of the patient attempting violent suicide (Åsberg et al. 1976), one wonders whether this is an indication of the severity of the depressed state and how this may help in the clinical management of the patients. There is no evidence to my knowledge that such patients are more resistant to therapy than those with only a slightly reduced, or even normal CSF 5-HIAA concentration. Furthermore, as Matussek emphasizes in his presentation, psychopaths with high aggression scores, but who were not depressed,

Pharmacology Department, University College, Galway, Ireland

Depressive Illness: Prediction of Course and Outcome
Edited by T. Helgason and R. J. Daly

were also found to have a low CSF 5-HIAA concentration (Brown et al. 1982).

The widespread use of the dexamethasone suppression test (DST) as a marker of depression undoubtedly makes this a robust test (Carroll et al. 1980) despite the "false positives" which may arise in the case of patients with senile dementia, alcoholism, and anorexia nervosa (Ballin et al. 1983). Whether the abnormal DST in such cases is due to secondary symptoms of depression or to such factors as an abnormal nutritional status (Carroll 1978) still awaits elucidation. Despite these disadvantages, the DST has been shown to be a useful state-dependent marker of major depressive disorder in that dexamethasone suppresses the elevated cortisol level in those patients responding to antidepressant therapy, but fails to do so in those who do not respond to treatment. Other neuroendocrine markers of depression and of response to treatment include the blunted thyroid-stimulating hormone response to thyroid-releasing hormone (Loosen and Prange 1980), a blunted growth hormone response to a variety of biogenic amine receptor agonists (Risch et al. 1981), and a blunted prolactin response to opiate receptor stimulation (Judd et al. 1982). While these tests of neuroendocrine function may help to establish the hypothesis that there is an abnormality in neurotransmitter function in the limbic system-hypothalamic region in depressed patients, there is little evidence to suggest that any of these tests are superior to the DST. Another possible explanation for the abnormal hormonal responses seen in the deprssed patient is that the changes in limbic-hypothalamic activity and receptor sensitivity might coincide with an alteration in the circadian rhythm of the patients (Wirz-Justice and Wehr 1983).

One of the most important developments in the search for biological markers of affective disorders in recent years has involved the study of changes in neurotransmitter receptor function on platelets and lymphocytes. It is well-established that tricyclic antidepressants inhibit the re-uptake of biogenic amines into both nerve terminals and platelets (Toddrick and Tait 1969). The platelet may be considered to be a model of the nerve terminal (Weiss 1975; Shaskin and Snyder 1970; Stahl and Meltzer 1978) and studies of the uptake of [^{3}H]serotonin and of the aggregation rate of a platelet-rich plasma in the presence of exogenous serotonin have been used to assess changes in serotonergic function in patients with depression. Most studies of the uptake of [^{3}H]serotonin in untreated depressed patients have reported a reduction in the transport rate (Coppen et al. 1978; Tuomisto et al. 1979; Scott 1979) that returns to control values following effective drug treatment (Tuomisto et al. 1979; Born et al. 1980; Healy et al. 1983). These findings suggest that the re-uptake of [^{3}H]serotonin by platelets can be used as a state-dependent marker of depression and as a marker of response to treatment. In this regard, it is of interest to find that the changes in the serotonin uptake rate are qualitatively similar for all kinds of antidepressant drugs irrespective of their presumed action on the serotonergic system as indicated by their effect on the uptake of [^{3}H]serotonin into synaptosomes prepared from rat brain following their acute administration. Furthermore, the duration of treatment required for the change in [^{3}H]serotonin uptake approximates to that needed for a clinical response to treatment to occur (i.e., approximately 2 weeks). The duration of drug treatment alone is not responsible for the normalization of serotonin reuptake, as the latter does not change in the absence of a clinical response (Healy et al. 1983).

While the mechanism whereby the normalization of [^{3}H]serotonin uptake occurs is unclear, it has been hypothesized that changes in receptor number, amine transport, and receptor function are correlated with an abnormal circadian rhythm in the depressed patient (Kafka 1980; Wirz-Justice and Campbell 1982). Effective antidepressant treatment may therefore lead to a correction of the circadian abnormality thereby returning amine transport and receptor function to normal. This hypothesis has been supported by the study of Healy et al. (1985) who showed that the [^{3}H]serotonin uptake into the platelets of untreated depressed patients at 0600 h, 0900 h, and 12 noon did not differ, whereas following effective antidepressant therapy the uptake rate at these times resembled the controls in that the rates were nearly twice as great at 0600 h, and 0900 h as at noon. Our studies have also shown that the serotonin-induced platelet aggregation rate was significantly reduced in the untreated depressive, but returned to normal following effective treatment (Healy et al. 1983). This finding helps to support the results reported by De Montigny and Aghajanian (1978) who showed that chronic antidepressant treatment increased the responsiveness of serotonin receptors in the rodent forebrain. Thus, the serotonin-induced platelet aggregation response, like the [^{3}H]serotonin uptake rate, may be considered a state marker for depression.

There is good experimental evidence to suggest that such tricyclic antidepressants as imipramine and desipramine bind specifically with high affinity to platelets and nerve terminals. Their binding sites are associated with, but not identical to, the active transport sites for serotonin and noradrenaline, respectively (Briley et al. 1979; Rehavi et al. 1981; Paul et al. 1981). There is evidence that the number of [^{3}H]imipramine binding sites on the platelet membrane of untreated depressed patients is reduced but, unlike the serotonin uptake rate, does not return to normal following effective treatment (Briley et al. 1980), thereby suggesting that this is a trait, rather than a state marker of depression. Whether the [^{3}H]imipramine binding sites on the platelet membrane may be considered as a genetic marker for depression still awaits elucidation.

In his presentation, Matussek summarizes the results of several studies on depressed patients in whom there is an apparent reduction in α-adrenergic receptor sensitivity. Much of the evidence preporting to show a reduction in α_2-adrenergic responsiveness is indirect and based upon changes in clonidine-induced neuroendocrine responses. The major problems regarding the specificity of such tests for depression have been discussed by Matussek et al. (1980; 1984). Direct determination of the density of α_2-adrenoceptors on platelets has been undertaken in several studies, but the results are equivocal, with some investigators showing an increase (Kafka et al. 1980; Garcia-Sevilla et al. 1981;

Healy et al. 1983), others a decrease (Wood and Coppen 1981), and still others no change (Stahl et al. 1983; Murphy et al. 1974). Following effective antidepressant treatment, the density of these receptors as assessed by various ^{3}H-ligand binding techniques, has been reported as largely decreased (Garcia-Sevilla et al. 1981; Healy et al. 1983) or unchanged (Stahl et al. 1983).

The differences reported in the various studies can, at least partially, be attributed to differences in the patient population studied. Those patients showing delusions (Nasr et al. 1981) or reactive depression (Pimoule et al. 1983; Healy et al. 1985) show no change in the density of α_2-receptor binding sites. It may be concluded that changes in α_2-receptor density may represent an epiphenomenon unrelated to the aetiology of the disease, but until detailed studies have been undertaken using a clinically homogeneous population of patients in which both the receptor density and function are assessed, any conclusions implicating an abnormality in α_2-receptor function in depression will remain equivocal. Some of the factors which may influence the changes in α_2-adrenoceptor functions on platelets have been reviewed by Elliott (1984). So far, only Wood and Coppen (1985) have attempted to assess changes in adrenoceptor function on platelets from depressed patients and shown that the aggregatory response to noradrenaline was decreased in the untreated depressive.

Few studies have been made of changes in β-adrenoceptor density or lymphocyte membranes prepared from depressed patients and the results of these limited studies are inconclusive. Thus, Pandey et al. (1979) and Extein et al. (1979) reported on decreased functional activity and receptor density while Shimuzu and Fujita (1981) and Healy et al. (1983) have shown that the receptor density is slightly increased in the untreated patients but returns to control value following effective treatment. There is evidence that the lymphocyte fractions used in these studies are heavily contaminated with platelets (Steer and Atlas 1982) which also contain β-adrenoceptors. This serves to emphasize the caution which must be exercised in extrapolating from changes in β-receptor density on lymphocytes to the presumed functional changes in the receptors in the brain of the depressed patient.

Despite the early seminal studies by Metalnikov (1934) on the role of the brain in modifying the anaphylactic response, knowledge of the specific brain regions which might be involved in immunoregulation is very limited. Lesions of the hypothalamus and the reticular formation have been shown by Jankovič and Izakovĭ (1973) to lead to a marked decrease in both humoral and cell-mediated immunity. As the hypothalamus-pituitary-adrenal axis is disturbed in depression, it might be anticipated that changes in immunoregulation might also occur in such patients. Such a view is consistent with epidemiological studies showing that the incidence of cancer is increased in depressed patients (Rogers et al. 1979), while other studies have shown that the stress of bereavement is often accompanied by an impairment of cell-mediated immunity (Bartrop et al. 1977).

More recently, Kronfol et al. (1983) compared the in vitro lymphocytic responses to three different mitogens in drug-free depressed patients compared to age- and sex-matched controls and observed a marked decrease in the lymphocytic mitogenic activity of the depressed group, thereby indicating an impairment in the cell-mediated immunity. In this study, there was evidence that the impairment was increased with the increasing severity of the illness. Other studies have shown that the IgG and IgM responses were significantly lower in depressed patients than their controls (Linn et al. 1982). However, in a study of the immunoglobulin profile in a group of drug-free depressed patients by O'Neill and Leonard (1986) no change could be detected even though all the patients had HAM-D scores >17. Linn et al. (1982) have suggested that the effect of stressful stimuli on the immune responsiveness may differ according to the severity of the depressed state which might explain the differences between the results of their studies. The rate at which lymphocytes engulf a chemiluminescent probe in vitro has also been investigated by O'Neill and Leonard (1986) in a group of depressed patients and their controls. In this study, the lymphocyte response was determined before and during drug treatment and the results clearly demonstrated that the activity of the lymphocytes was significantly decreased before the commencement of treatment, but returned to control values in those patients who responded to drug treatments. This suggests that the lymphocyte chemotaxis test may be useful as a state-dependent marker of depression; preliminary data suggest that the lymphocyte responsiveness in alcoholics and senile dementia patients does not differ appreciably from nondepressed patients.

Clearly more extensive studies must be undertaken to validate such findings, but these preliminary studies serve to emphasize the interaction between genetic, immune, neuroendocrine, and behavioural changes in depressed patients. Such studies also indicate that depression is a disease which affects physiological processes throughout the body and is not confined to an abnormality in central neurotransmission.

Conclusion

The lack of reproducibility of the biochemical changes found by different investigators studying biological markers of depression may be ascribed to such factors as the heterogeneous nature of the patient population studied, imprecise diagnostic criteria being applied, too small a patient sample size, nonstandardisation of the assay methods used, failure to take into account the effect of changes in circadian rhythm and the effects of diet and exercise on the parameters being determined. Until research protocols are designed which take such factors into account, it seems unlikely that any major advance in our understanding of the aetiology of affective disorders and of predictors of response to treatment will be obtained.

Matussek has critically assessed the major areas for biological research which need to be considered in future and, in my view, correctly argued for the need for multicentred, multidisciplinary studies to be performed using rigidly observed protocols. While there are an inordinate number of questions that need to be answered in this area of biological psychiatry, the following questions may help to focus the interest of researchers onto some of the areas in which a search for biological markers may prove to be particularly valuable:

1. Assess the usefulness of the [^{3}H]serotonin uptake rate into platelets as a state-dependent marker of depression. Could this test prove to be as useful diagnostically as the DST?
2. Study platelet [^{3}H]imipramine binding in depressed patients and their near relatives to see if such data can be used to select those individuals who are predisposed to depression.
3. Assess changes in cortical evoked potentials, REM sleep latency, and cognitive function in depressed patients before and following treatment to see whether such psychophysiological variables can be correlated with the data obtained from the platelet studies.
4. Investigate the biological phenomena which may be indirectly correlated with changes in neurotransmission in the depressed patient in an attempt to broaden the basis of the conceptually restrictive "amine hypothesis" of depression. Changes in electrolyte flux (e.g., Ca, Na, K) across erythrocyte and lymphocyte membranes, and factors governing the changes in lymphocyte mobility, may help to lay the basis for a more holistic approach to the biology of depression.
5. Profile the changes in neurotransmitter function in the platelets, lymphocytes and erythrocytes of well-defined subgroups of depressed patients (e.g., therapy-resistant depressives; agoraphobics and "atypical" depressives who appear to respond to antidepressant treatment; senile dements with depression) and compare these with patients with endogenous depression. In this way it might be possible to determine which biochemical parameter(s) acts as a marker of the main symptoms of depression and which may correlate better with the secondary symptoms of the illness.

The search for the "black bile" has eluded investigators for 2000 years. Perhaps one of the reasons for this has been because the questions asked have been too advanced for the technology needed to answer them. With the advent of sensitive and reliable biochemical and psychophysiological techniques, the time may have come to determine the identity of the "black bile" which is responsible for untold suffering in 5% of the population.

References

Åsberg M, Thoren P, Traskman L, Bertilsson L, Ringleergern N (1976) Serotonin depression: a biochemical sub-group within the affective disorders. Science 191:478–479

Ballin J, Gottfries C-G, Karlsson I (1983) Dexamethasone suppression test and serum prolactin in dementia disorders. Br J Psychiatry 143:277–278

Bartrop RW, Lazarus L, Luckhurst E, Kiloh LG, Penny R (1977) Depressed lymphocyte function after bereavement. Lancet I:884–886

Born GVR, Gragnani G, Martin K (1980) Long-term effects of lithium on the uptake of 5-hydroxytryptamine by human platelets. Br J Clin Pharmacol 8:321–326

Brown GM, Ebert MH, Goyer PF, Jimerson DC, Klein WJ, Bunney WE, Goodwin FK (1982) Aggression, suicide and serotonin: relationships to CSF amine metabolites. Am J Psychiatry 139:741–746

Briley MS, Raisman R, Langer SZ (1979) Human platelets possess high affinity binding sites for ^{3}H-imipramine. Eur J Pharmacol 58:347–348

Briley MS, Langer SZ, Raisman R, Sechter D, Zarifian E (1980) ^{3}H-Imipramine binding sites are decreased in platelets of untreated depressed patients. Science 303:1209–1210

Carroll BJ (1978) Neuroendocrine function in psychiatric disorders. In: Lipton MA, Di Maschio A, Killam KF (eds) Psychopharmacology: a generation of progress. Raven, New York, pp 487–497

Carroll BJ, Feinberg M, Steiner M, Haskett RF, James N, Tarika J (1980). Diagnostic application of the dexamethasone suppression test in depressed outpatients. Adv Biol Psychiatry 5:107–116

Coppen A, Swade C, Wood K (1978). Platelet 5-hydroxytryptamine accummulation in depressive illness. Clin Chim Acta 87:165–168

De Montigny C, Aghajanian GK (1978) Tricyclic antidepressants: long-term treatment increases responsivity of rat forebrain neurons to serotonin. Science 202:1310–1306

Elliott JM (1984) Platelet receptor binding studies in affective disorders. J Affective Disord 6:219–239

Extein I, Tallman J, Smith CC (1979) Changes in lymphocyte beta adrenergic receptors in depression and mania. Psychiatry Res 1:191–197

Garcia-Seville JA, Zis AP, Zelnick JC, Smith CB (1981) Tricyclic antidepressant treatment decreases α_2-adrenoceptors on human platelet membranes. Eur J Pharmacol 69:121–123

Healy D, Carney PA, Leonard BE (1983) Monoamine related markers of depression: changes following treatment. J Psychiatr Res 17:251–260

Healy D, Carney PA, Leonard BE (1985) Circadian abnormalities in 5-HT uptake in depression. In: Redfern PA, Campbell IC, Davies JA, Martin KF (eds) Circadian rhythms in the central nervous system. MacMillan, London

Jankovič DA, Isakovič K (1973) Neuroendocrine correlates of immune response. Int Arch Allergy 45:360–372

Judd LL, Risch SC, Parker DC, Janowsky DS, Segal DS, Huey LY (1982) The effect of a methadone challenge on the prolactin and growth hormone responses of psychiatric patients and normal controls. Psychopharmac Bull 18:204–212

Kafka MS, van Kammen DP, Kleinman JE (1980) Alpha adrenergic receptor function in schizoprenia, affective disorders and some neurological diseases. Comm Psychopharmacol 4:477–486

Kafka MS, Wirz-Justice A, Naber D, Marangos PJ, O'Donohue TL, Wehr A (1982) The effect of lithium on circadian neurotransmitter receptor rhythms. Neuropsychobiology 8:41–50

Kronfol Z, Silva J, Greden J, Dembinski S, Gardner R, Carroll B (1983) Impaired lymphocyte function in depressive illness. Life Sci 33:241–247

Leonard BE (1982) Current status of the biogenic amine theory of depression. Neurochem Int 4:339–350

Linn BS, Linn MW, Jensen J (1982) Degree of depression and immune responsiveness. Psychosom Med 44:128–129
Loosen PT, Prange AJ (1980) Thyrotropin-releasing hormone (TRH): a useful tool for psychoneuroendocrine investigation. Psychoneuroendocrinology 5:63–80
Matussek N, Ackenheil M, Hippius HT, Müller F, Schröder H-T, Schultes H, Wasilewski B (1980) Effect of clonidine on growth hormone release in psychiatric patients and controls. Psychiatr Res 2:25–36
Matussek N, Ackenheil M, Herz M (1984) The dependence of the clonidine growth hormone test on alcohol drinking habits and the menstrual cycle. Psychoneuroendocrinology 9:173–177
Metalnikov S (1934) Rôle du système nerveux et des facteurs biologiques et psychiques dans l'immunité. Masson, Paris
Montgomery SA (1982) The non-selective effect of selective antidepressants. Adv Biochem Psychopharmac 31:49–56
Murphy DL, Donnelly C, Moskowitz J (1974) Catecholamine receptor function in depressed patients. Am J Psychiatry 131:1389–1391
Nasr S, Daiguji M, Tang C, Meltzer HY (1980) Comparison of midday serum dopamine-β-hydroxylase activity in depressed patients and normal controls. Commun Psychopharmacol 4(4):263–267
O'Neill B, Leonard BE (1986) Is there an abnormality in neutrophil phagocytosis in depression? IRCS Med Sci, 14:802–803
Pandey GN, Pysken MW, Garter DL, Davis JM (1979) Beta-adrenergic receptor function in affective illness. Am J Psychiatry 136:675–678
Paul SM, Rehavi M, Rice KC (1981) Does high affinity ^{3}H-imipramine binding label serotonin re-uptake sites in brain and platelets? Life Sci 28:2753–2760
Pimoule C, Briley MS, Gay C, Loo H, Sechter D, Zarifian E, Raisman R, Langer SZ (1983) ^{3}H-Rauwolscine binding in platelets from depressed patients and healthy volunteers. Psychopharmacology 79:398–402
Rehavi M, Skolnick P, Hulihan B, Paul SM (1981) High affinity binding of ^{3}H-desipramine to rat cerebral cortex: relationship to tricyclic antidepressant induced inhibition of noradrenaline uptake. Eur J Pharmacol 70:597–603
Risch SC, Kalin NH, Murphy DL (1981) Pharmacological challenge strategies: implications for neurobehavioural mechanisms in affective disorders and treatment approaches. J Clin Pharmacol 1:238–245
Rogers MP, Dubey D, Reich P (1979) The influence of the psyche and the brain on immunity and disease susceptibility: a critical review. Psychosom Med 41:147–164
Sacchetti E, Maria E, Negri F, Biondi PA, Smeraldi E, Cazzullo CL (1979) 3-Methoxy-4-hydroxyphenylglycol and primary depression: clinical and pharmacological considerations. Biol Psychiatry 14:473–484
Schildkraut JJ, Orsulak PJ, Schatzberg AF (1978) Towards a biochemical classification of depressive disorders. 1. Differences in urinary excretion of MHPG and other catecholamine metabolites in clinically defined sub-types of depression. Arch Gen Psychiatr 35:1427–1433
Scott M, Reading HW, Loudon TB (1979) Studies on human blood platelets in affective disorder. Psychopharmacology 60:131–135
Shaskin EG, Snyder SJ (1970) Kinetics of serotonin accumulation into slices from rat brain: relationship to catecholamine uptake. J Pharmacol Exp Therap 175:404–418
Shimuzu T, Fujita M (1981) Effect of β-adrenergic receptor blocking agents in depression as measured by plasma noradrenaline concentrations and blood pressure. In: Langer S (ed) New vistas in depression. Pergamon, New York, 126–134
Stahl SM, Meltzer HY (1978) A kinetic and pharmacologic analysis of 5-hydroxytryptamine transport by human platelets and platelet storage granules. Comparison and central serotonergic neurons. J Pharmacol Exp Therap 205:118–121
Stahl SM, Lenocine PM, Ciaranello RD (1983) Platelet alpha$_2$ adrenergic receptor sensitivity in major depressive disorder. Psychiatr Res 10:157–164

Steer ML, Atlas D (1982) Demonstration of human platelet β-adrenergic receptor using I^{125}-labelled cyano pindolol and I^{125}-labelled hydroxy benzyl pindolol. Biochem Biophys Acta 686:240–244

Todrick A, Tait AC (1969) The inhibition of human platelet 5-hydroxytryptamine uptake by tricyclic antidepressive drugs. The relation between structure and potency. J Pharm Pharmacol 21:751–762

Tuomisto T, Tukiainen E, Ahlfors UG (1979) Decreased uptake of 5-hydroxytryptamine in blood platelets from patients with endogenous depression. Psychopharmacology 65:141–147

Van Praag H, De Hahn S (1979) Central serotonin metabolism and frequency of depression. Psychiatry Res 1:219–224

Veith RC, Bielski RJ, Bloom V (1983) Urinary MHPG excretion and treatment with desipramine and amitriptyline. J Clin Psychopharmacol 3:18–27

Weiss JJ (1975) Platelet physiology and abnormalities of platelet function. N Engl J Med 293:531–541

Wirz-Justice A, Campbell IC (1982) Antidepressant drugs can slow or dissociate circadian rhythms. Experientia 38:1301–1309

Wirz-Justice A, Wehr TA (1983) Neuropsychopharmacology and biological rhythms. Adv Biol Psychiatry 11:20–34

Wood K, Coppen A (1981) Platelet alpha-adrenoceptor sensitivity in depressive illness. Adv Biol Psychiatry 7:85–89

Wood K, Coppen A (1985) Platelet transport and receptor sites in depressive illness. In: Iversen SD (ed) Psychopharmacology: recent advances and future prospects. Oxford University Press, Oxford, pp 21–32

Image of Depression *

R. ÖHMAN, A. FRANCK HOLMKVIST, and S. NIELZÉN

Introduction

A depressive syndrome with its typical association of psychomotor retardation, anxiety, distortion of mood, disillusionment regarding the future, and lack of self-confidence with guilt feelings, is well-known to the medical profession. For the psychiatrist it is evident that the depressive syndromes reflect a multitude of mental disorders where, as in all other fields of medicine, a variety of background factors may be assigned etiological or symptomatological importance. The layman's insight and convictions on the relationships between etiology and depressive mood disorders are, however, often very distant from the physiological realities reflected by clinical experience and research in the field. It is therefore urged that our image of depression involve a search for biological correlates to this group of disorders. Whatever pathogenic factors may be imagined in the individual case, the biopathological process remains the crossroads for diagnostic and basic therapeutic work.

The unfortunately erroneous coupling of negative experiences with the general cause of pathological depression of mood may be understandable, but inhibits by prejudice rational collaborative research. Prevailing attitudes during the 1970s concerning depressive disorders, with sometimes uncritical acceptance of psychodynamic reasoning, created an unfortunate distance between the most flourishing period of neurobiological research and its clinical field of future application. During recent years a new generation of scientists, trained both clinically and in basic research have gained new momentum in biological psychiatry. The availability of new research tools has during this period enabled us to focus our image of depression on matrices of metabolism, regulation of energy, and electrophysiological events as patterns in a landscape where brain imaging techniques describe the exact topography down to its most minute coordinates. The biological research in depressive disorders has presented astonishing potential for interdisciplinary studies, both in the US and in Europe.

* The present study was supported by the Swedish Medical Research Foundation, project no. 4803
Department of Psychiatry, University Hospital, S-22185 Lund

Brain Imaging

The biological correlates of psychopathology and character were looked for, as early as Hippocrates, in body fluids and in organs, notably in the case of hysteria. Electrophysiological observations by Galvani (1737–1798), Albrecht von Haller (1707–1777), Sherrington (1857–1952), and Broca (1824–1880) successively convinced the medical profession that brain functions have central correlates to neurological but also to psychiatric disorders. Astonishingly this obvious fact has not yet been absorbed by many influential persons and notably not generally by laymen. The functional topography of the brain was revealed during the middle of the nineteenth century by Gustav Fritsch (1838–1927), Edward Hitzig (1838–1907), Wernicke (1848–1905), and others. Research primarily inspired by Jackson (1835–1911), Duchenne (1806–1875), and Charcot (1825–1893) superimposed the concept of the functional hierarchy and levels of the central nervous system. Successively, the gross anatomical image of the brain has been completed with perspectives on the organization of the cellular layers and neurotransmission, and with functional aspects of energy provision, transport, and recognition. All these are facets of the dynamic image of brain structure. Recent developments in the engineering of radiation detection and in computer technology have led to the development of new families of techniques devised to provide images of the living brain in a concrete sense. Computer tomography (CT), positron emission tomography (PET scanning), nuclear magnetic resonance (NMR), and three-dimensional regional cerebral blood flow (rCBF), all belong to the same family of technology. The potential of these methods in research and clinical evaluation of depressive states will be outlined below.

The Image of an Image

Since the topic is imaging techniques, it would be interesting at first to look at how clinical psychiatry successively built up its image of depression, how its image has been perceived. The visual image was always the cornerstone in the description of the patient. The artistic image of the mentally ill became successively a principle of diagnostic approach to psychiatric disorders. The diagnostic approach was the visual image as recognized in the old textbooks of psychiatry. Pinel (1745–1826), Charcot (1825–1893), and Kraepelin (1856–1926) taught psychiatry against the background of the immediate visual image of the patient – the face, posture, movements. Successively textbooks have changed their appearance, and today they contain facts or fictions, but not even with an appendix of patient histories and definitely without pictures conveying the image. However, the introduction of videotapes lately has in an even more powerful way enabled us to convey the visual description.

If we accept that affective disorders and psychopathology at large ultimately must have correlates to energy or structure-related processes in the central nervous system, we have to approach with a great scientific curiosity the new imaging techniques for CNS function and structure presently brought to us through the neurosciences.

Which are the most relevant and reliable techniques? Which findings are valid and how confusing are the artifacts? Future research work and clinical experience will give answers to these and similar questions. Presently it is somewhat like the blind fakirs "seeing the elephant, each differently interpreting the feeling of the tiny bit of the elephant that his hands can feel." Nelson Goodman (1982) states in "The way the world ist": "We cannot find out much about the way the world is by asking about the best or most faithful or most realistic way of seeing or picturing it. For the ways of seeing and picturing are many and various; strong, effective, useful, intriguing, or sensitive; others are weak, foolish, dull, or blurred. But even if all the latter are excluded, still none of the rest can lay any good claim to be the way of seeing or picturing the world the way it is." This also goes for affective disorders and imaging technique.

With this background, a brief survey will be given of some of the new imaging techniques of brain structure and function. Intentionally the technological principles are described only superficially as they may be more profoundly penetrated by consulting the literature in the field. This presentation is rather to be devoted to potential applications. The techniques may be used in understanding pathophysiology or for diagnostic recognition of affective disorders. At this stage of development interpretations of findings must be cautiously done by scientists from different fields. It has to be taken into account that the new technology on the one hand offers the opportunity of receiving the instant structure – a "frozen" image – and on the other it has the potential of dynamic reflection of brain function.

Cerebral Computer Tomography

Conventional X-ray images, with or without application of gas or radioopaque contrast, was for a number of years the only way of imaging the central nervous system in a patient. Although helpful in the recognition of gross structural malformation of cortical structures, ventricles, and vessles, its use in the diagnosis of affective disorders was only to exclude "organic processes of the CNS." The advent of CT, which had a tremendous impact on neuroradiology, did, however, contribute little to the diagnosis of affective states except the obvious and welcome relief of discomfort at investigation.

The introduction of the rotating scanner and computer application for image reconstruction, however, precipitated advancement in many related areas of research. The perfection of these methods is founded on the mathematical principle underlying image reconstruction resolved as a theoretical problem by Radon already in 1917. Of course the CT technique has been made practically usable only through advances in computer technology in recent years. Although a method with high resolution power (0.8 mm), its main purpose is for structural studies, for a "frozen" image (Margulis et al. 1983; Gwan Go et al. 1983).

Nuclear Magnetic Resonance (NMR)

Magnetism is a result of movements by electric charges. Electrons create such magnetic properties by orbital movements. Also the elements of the nucleus, protons and neutrons, have charges. The proton is positively charged and the neutron has an inhomogeneous composition of subparticles. Therefore, nuclear magnetic fields originate from such particles in motion. Paired particles eliminate the dipole structure while unpaired odd protons by rotation strengthen the dipole characteristic. Many isotopes like ^{1}H, ^{13}C, ^{15}N, ^{23}Na, and ^{31}P have such properties. When applying an external magnetic field, nuclear dipoles align themselves in the field. Transmitted electromagnetic radiation, radiowaves, can create resonance in the nuclear structure, causing transitions between different natural states of the system. When they return to equilibrium they will again emit radiation. By variations of magnetic field or energy of excitation, different principles for detecting nuclear magnetic structures can be constructed. We can listen to the signals from hydrogen or from other specific isotopes. By applying imaging techniques (NMR) similar to those of CT, these signals can be located and used in building a picture of the investigated tissue in any chosen plane.

The NMR methods presently available provide images of the brain that in contrast and resolution surpass any other technique. NMR does not utilize ionizing radiation and is, with due safety precautions, as yet considered harmless to tissue. Its contrast can be further enhanced by the administration of certain compounds. Specific studies of blood-brain-barrier function or cerebral blood flow or metabolism are thus possible. The present use of the method is directed towards structural studies. No conclusive investigations have so far been done on affective disorders.

The method has, however, a tremendous potential of development through which metabolic processes, energy levels, and receptor functions of the brain can be truly reflected.

Cerebral Blood Flow (CBF)

The cortical areas and nuclear structures consume for energy purposes large amounts of glucose and oxygen. The activity-related metabolism regulates the local blood flow. Regional cerebral blood flow thus mirrors regional cerebral activity.

The uptake and clearence of ^{133}Xenon is directly related to regional blood flow and thus becomes a tool for imaging cortical activity. The clinical application by Lassen and Ingvar with intracarotid injection and by Obrist and Risberg for inhalation of xenon, have lately been most helpful diagnostic tools in psychiatry. Dementias and vascular disorders can be recognized through specific flow patterns. The image of brain work at perception and activation using problem-solving tests has been valuable in the understanding of the interaction of different cortical areas. Continuing studies have demonstrated that psychotic patients have reduced frontal metabolism and that depressed states with anxiety may clearly increase the rate of CBF. The degree of anxiety can be visualized. On the other hand, depression without anxiety has been shown to be related to decreased rate of cerebral blood flow, especially in the dominant hemisphere (Lassen and Ingvar 1972; Obrist et al. 1975; Risberg et al. 1975; Silfverskiöld et al. 1985).

Positron Emission Tomography (PET)

PET is one of the most exciting developments in imaging techniques. It is probably never used as a routine diagnostic instrumentation but a typical research tool in neurobiology.

Radionuclides such as ^{11}C, ^{13}N, ^{15}O, and ^{18}F are positron emittors, that can be generated by radiation in a cyclotron accelerator. Although having very short half-lives, they can be included in synthetic procedures and introduced as labels in an array of compounds, amino acids, sugars, and drugs, for the study of metabolism, transport, receptor mechanisms, etc. Such compounds introduced into the CNS emit positrons and can thereby be located in a tomographic fashion with a resolution of around 2–3 mm. Such equipment is so far very complex – but push button laboratories are soon to be on the market. With the use of labelled drugs, receptor sites and densities can be located. The use of ^{18}F deoxyglucose has enabled metabolic studies that also include affective disorders, although the results are so far preliminary and report limited numbers of cases. The most convincing studies have been performed by Mazziotta and collaborators in Los Angeles. Judged from the impressive clinical protocols, extensive efforts have been made in diagnosing and evaluating the clinical sample.

Among the findings communicated in summary (Baxter et al. 1985) the following are noted: Bipolar patients in a depressive state had a significantly lower supratentorial metabolic rate ($P<0.001$) than reference individuals. Normals, unipolar depressed, and bipolar hypomanic patients showed no significant differences in group comparisons. Clinical improvement in depressed bipolars is associated with normalization of metabolism. Rapid cycling bipolars showed large changes of metabolism, even within 24 h. A subset of unipolar depressed patients, not distinguishable on clinical grounds, showed lower glucose metabolic rate in the left lateral inferior frontal cortex. Patients with unipolar depressions showed a significant decrease of the caudate nucleus/hemispheric metabolic ratio ($P<0.01$).

In earlier studies Buchsbaum et al. (1984) reported similar results, i.e., a decreased rate of regional cerebral glucose metabolism in affective illness.

The results, interpreted with caution, suggest that further studies of affective states may be very rewarding in illuminating different pathophysiological subtypes of affective disorders (Buchsbaum et al. 1984; Phelps et al. 1984; Baxter et al. 1985; Crow 1982).

Electroencephalography (EEG)

Modern computer techniques have also revived EEG. Frequency analysis and displays for imaging have made the registrations more comprehensive and permit numerical handling. Developments in the field of evoked electroencephalographic responses to stimuli have made it possible to study in greater detail deviations in perception among psychiatric patients. Computerization of the registration and displays with subtraction of normal background patterns may lead to even more sophisticated use of EEG, probably also in affective disorders where perceptual processes are significantly distorted (Morstyn et al. 1983).

Concluding Remarks

As already pointed out, there is in psychiatry a long tradition of founding the diagnosis also on the visual observation of the patient. This visual aspect of diagnosis has fortunately not completely vanished from the contemporary scene. Freud (1856–1939) largely rejected the importance of seeing and observing the patient and emphasized psychoanalysis as a process of listening. He taught psychiatrists to use the "third ear," and the auditive channel became the major instrument for diagnosis and imaging the unconscious material in the patient.

The new imaging techniques, presently being developed by modern technology, again strenghen the clinician's visual perception of the mental process and psychopathology. Technology has in fact provided psychiatrists with a kind of "third eye" to be employed when searching for new vistas in diagnostic and therapeutic work.

References

Baxter LR, Maziotta JC, Phelps ME, Schwartz JM, Gerner RH (1985) Local cerebral glucose metabolism in affective disorders. Brain 85:303–307 (Abstract)

Buchsbaum MS, Cappelletti J, Ball R, Hazlett E, King AC, Johnson J, Wu J, DeLisi LE (1984) Positron emission tomographic image measurement in schizophrenia and affective disorders. Ann Neurol (Suppl) 15:157–165

Crow TJ (ed) (1982) Disorders of neurohumoural transmission. Academic, London
Goodman N (1982) On thoughts without words. Cognition 12(2):211–217
Gwan Go K, van Dijk P, Luiten AL, Brouwer-van Herwijnen AA, van der Leeuw LCL, Kamman RL, Vencken LM, Wilmink J, Berendsen HJC (1983) Interpretation of nuclear magnetic resonance tomograms of the brain. J Neurosurg 59:574–584
Lassen NA, Ingvar DH (1972) Radioisotopic assessment of regional cerebral blood flow. Prog Nucl Med 1:376–409
Margulis AR, Higgins CB, Kaufman L, Crooks LE (eds) (1983) Clinical magnetic resonance imaging. Radiology Research and Education Foundation
Morstyn R, Duffy FH, McCarley RW (1983) Altered topography of EEG spectral content in schizophrenia. Electr Clin Neurophys 56:263–271
Obrist WD, Thompson HK, Wang HS, Wilkinson WE (1975) Regional blood flow estimated by ^{133}Xenon inhalation. Stroke 6:245–256
Phelps ME, Maziotta JC, Baxter L, Gerner R (1984) Positron emission tomographic study of affective disorders: problems and strategies. Ann Neurol (Suppl) 15:149–156
Risberg J, Ali Z, Wilson EM, Wills EL, Halsey JH (1975) Regional cerebral blood flow by ^{133}Xenon inhalation. Preliminary evaluation of an initial slope index in patients with unstable flow compartments. Stroke 6:142–148
Silverskiöld P, Gustafson L, Risberg J, Rosén I (1985) EEG and rCBF related to clinical outcome: acute and late effects. J Cereb Blood Flow Metab 5 [Suppl 1]:187–188

Physical Ill-Health, Age and Depression

J. R. M. COPELAND

The Prevalence and Outcome of Depression in Old Age

The prevalence of disease can only be assessed by community studies. Such studies of depression are fraught with the difficulties of defining not only the limits of illness but also the diagnostic criteria to be used. As a result it is difficult to compare the results of the various studies which have been done on samples of elderly subjects. Most workers have attempted to distinguish two types of depression. Although they are variously named, the divisions broadly adopted can be equated with severe and minor illness. From the first major study to examine a random sample of elderly community subjects by Kay et al. (1964), to our own investigations (Copeland et al. 1987a), the reported prevalence of severe or major depression has varied only between 1.0%–4.0%, which is perhaps a surprising degree of agreement given the diverse criteria used (Weissman and Myers 1980; Persson 1980; Blazer and Williams 1980; Blazer 1982; Cooper and Schwartz 1982; Gurland et al. 1983; Kay et al. 1985; Copeland et al. 1987a, b). The prevalance of minor depression has varied rather more widely between studies. This is not surprising as defining the limits of illness and normal behaviour are additional problems which bedevil the study of neurotic conditions. It also seems possible that the levels of minor depression may truly vary between populations. In our study we used standardized semistructured methods for assessing mental state, the Geriatric Mental State (GMS) AGECAT Package, and a computer diagnostic system (Copeland et al. 1986). We were able to show that the levels of depression as a whole, in both New York and London were similar at 16.2% for the former and 19.4% for the latter (Copeland et al. 1987b), whereas the level in a sample drawn from a rural area of the United Kingdom, using the same method, was substantially less, at 9.5% (Copeland et al. 1988). It had been expected that, at least the level of reactive, minor or neurotic depression would have been higher in New York where life, at the time of the study, was shown to be more difficult and dangerous for old people, and adverse life events presumed to be more frequent. The reason it was not is not clear, and requires more investigation. It may have been due to lower expectations among the New York el-

University Department of Psychiatry, Royal Liverpool Hospital, PO Box 147, Liverpool L693 Bx, United Kingdom

Depressive Illness: Prediction of Course and Outcome
Edited by T. Helgason and R. J. Daly

derly, 60% of whom had been immigrants. The association with expressed physical symptoms elicited by enquiry, was also higher in New York where access to medical services was more difficult for elderly persons, but again this did not seem to result in either a greater prevalence or severity of depression as a whole in that city. The prevalence of depression requiring intervention in younger age groups had been assessed by Brown and Harris (1978) on a random sample of women aged 19–59, as about 16%. Therefore, there seems little evidence that depression as a whole is more prevalent among older than among younger populations.

The age patterns for depression by half decade in our samples were roughly similar in both New York and London, that for depressed males showing a fall in the rate at ages 70–74 and higher rates in older age groups, while that characteristic of depressed females showed higher rates between 65 and 74 than at 75 years and over. Reasons for this are not clear. The association with physical illness is discussed later. One possibility which must be considered is the selective death of depressed males between ages 70 and 74. Kay and Bergmann (1966) in their follow-up study had commented on such a finding. Our own longitudinal study of depressed elderly community subjects in Liverpool also found an increased death rate in depressed persons as high as 27% over 3 years, compared to 16% for nondepressed subjects. The majority of deaths were among depressed males. More studies are required which should pay particular attention to the influence of physical illness and its severity, and to past, personal and family history of depression, in order to gain insight into depression during the full life span.

Analysis of the rural sample which is on-going at present, suggests a much lower level of depression than for the urban samples, probably accounted for by a lower rate of adverse life events as assessed by the Bedford College (London) method, adapted for use with elderly subjects.

Post (1951) and Roth and Morrissey (1952) were the first to distinguish the comparatively hopeful outcome of depressed subjects from the outcome of those suffering from organic disorders. Kay and Bergmann (1966) re-examined a random community sample of 297 persons originally aged 65 and over, 4 years after their cross-sectional study. They found that for those developing functional disorders, which included both neuroses and psychoses, during the 4-year period, the predictors of onset were anxiety symptoms, physical disability, and depressive symptoms. Nielsen et al. in the Samsø study (1977), appeared to show that subjects with functional psychoses and neuroses had patterns of survival not dissimilar from normal subjects.

Murphy (1983) undertook a prospective study of 124 subjects aged 65 and over who had consulted the hospital services for the first time. She followed up the subjects 1 year later using Feighner et al.'s (1972) criteria for depression and standardized interviews including the Bedford College method for describing adverse life events. Only one-third of the group was found to have had a good outcome. Poor outcome was associated with severe initial illness especially the presence of depressive delusions, physical health problems and severe life events during the follow-up year. This careful study showed therefore, that the prognosis of depression sufficiently severe to be referred to hospital, had a much poorer outcome in the elderly than had previously been supposed. Copeland et al., on the basis of their longitudinal study in Liverpool, found the outcome for the depressed in the community somewhat similar, even though there were fewer severe illnesses in this setting. In the analysis so far, after 3 years, 27.1% of those suffering from depression had died, 30.0% had made a full recovery, and 42.9% were still regarded as depressed by the interviewing psychiatrists.

In order to discover the true prevalence of serious depression and to be able to divide this into bipolar, unipolar, early, and late onset depressions, it will be necessary to mount population studies running into several thousands of subjects or to be able to pool the results of several studies. Before this can be achieved, standardized methods of assessment, including mental state, historical, family and informant information must be fully developed and gain wide acceptance. A method of standardizing diagnosis which eliminates observer variability is also required. Work is going ahead on these problems and some comparisons can already be made between computer-generated diagnoses for elderly subjects. The GMS AGECAT Package is one such attempt. Although a number of centres are collaborating in this work, it must be extended if more specific issues are to be addressed. A further advantage of standardized methods of diagnosis, is that, with adequate training and checks of reliability nonmedical raters can replace costly medical staff for ordinary data collection. In any case more stringent criteria are required for identfying major and minor depressive illness. Striking differences have been claimed for the prevalence rates of quite severe depression between centres when using the same (DSM III; American Psychiatric Association 1980) criteria to identify major affective disorder in elderly persons.

Physical Illness and Depression

There is general agreement that the division between mind and body is no longer tenable. However, even if we adopt the view that they are inseparable, it is nevertheless convenient clinically to regard them as two functions constantly interacting. Thus, all disease may be seen to lie on a continuum between almost pure physical illness and almost pure psychiatric illness. Diagnostic difficulties arise because many medical doctors still tend to behave as if they believed in Descartes' myth and ignore what they perceive as the nondominant disease. Many patients do likewise, consciously or unconsciously denying one set of symptoms, usually but not always the psychological ones.

Many studies now present overwhelming evidence that physical and psychiatric illnesses coexist to a greater extent than can be accounted for by chance. Morris (1962) emphasized the proportion of physical illness amongst new admissions to a mental hospital. Gibson (1961) showed that 62% of admissions for affective disorder had physical illness which ought not to have been ignored. For those aged over 65 the proportion was even higher. Kay et al. (1964) reported that 41% of the elderly functionally ill in a random community sample had moderate to severe physical illness. Koranyi (1980), reviewing studies of 4000 psychiatric patients published between 1937 and 1979 found that about one-half the patients were said to have had a coexistent major medical illness, at least one-half again unrecognised. Copeland and Gurland (1978) using semistructured interview techniques to examine patients aged over 65 admitted to a variety of hospitals, identified 39% of those entering a psychiatric hospital as suffering from affective disorders, in a geriatric hospital the proportion was 15%, in a geriatric day hospital 30% and on the general medical wards 31%.

The correlation of depression with physical illness in the community studies was high, 0.47 in New York and 0.37 in London (Gurland et al. 1983). Correlations above 0.08 were significant at the 0.05 level. The age patterns for depression in both sexes were similar to those for physical illness; the one appearing to mirror the other.

Physical Illness as a Likely Cause of Depression

First, there are the acute and chronic brain disorders in which physical illness may act on the brain directly as in tumours, stroke and multiple sclerosis, or indirectly as in endocrine disorders, dietary deficiencles, anaemia, drugs, etc.

Moffic and Paykel (1975) judged that in a sample of medical inpatients, 65% of cases of depression were reactive to the physical illness, varying with its severity. In a further 21% the depression appeared to have preceded the physical illness, and in 14% the somatic features of depression had simply been mistaken by the medical personnel for physical illness.

Kramlinger et al. (1983) found 25% of admissions to a chronic pain clinic had definite depression, mainly of the reactive type.

Mann et al. (1984) found depression in residential homes particularly associated with visual handicap and incontinence. Bukberg et al. (1984) found 42% of cancer patients met the criteria for major depressive disorder. In our London community study, depression was found to be associated with restriction of mobility within the home, due to physical disability.

Parkinson's disease illustrates some of the complexities encountered in making a diagnosis of depression in the presence of physical illness and determining its cause. Here the symptoms of the disease itself may mimic depression. Depression may be reactive to the physical disease or related to medication. Both conditions may require treatment.

Lloyd (1977) reviewed the factors which appeared to determine a psychological reaction to physical illness. He commented on the severity of the latter, the personality of the patient and his or her coping strategies, and the response of the society to the illness.

Depression may modify the course of physical illness. Querido (1959) studied 1630 general hospital inpatients and found their "distress" a better predictor of prognosis than the judgement of the clinicians. Rutter (1963) found anxiety and depression better predictors of the outcome of peptic ulceration than the clinical features and course of the disease itself. Others have postulated similar findings for myocardial infarction. It is possible that depression influences patient's compliance or adversely affects cardiac and respiratory performance.

Physical illness may modify the course of depression. As we have already noted, Murphy (1983) followed up 124 elderly first attenders for depression. One year later she found that chronic physical ill-health was one of the problems most likely to determine a poor outcome.

Depression as a Possible Cause of Physical Illness

The case for depression as a causal factor in physical illness is less well established. Bereavement is reported to be associated with a higher mortality rate, perhaps through its effects on the cardiovascular system. Heine and Sainsbury in 1970 had postulated that repeated episodes of depression with anxiety and agitation led to sustained rise in blood pressure. Adverse life events have been shown to precede some cases of myocardial infarction (Connolly 1976) as well as depression. Murphy and Brown (1980) claimed from their studies that adverse life events in themselves did not predispose to physical illness unless they were also the cause of an acute psychiatric reaction. Brown and Harris (1978) found a small increased risk of physical illness in subjects with depression not preceded by significant life events.

Many authors report the tendency of the elderly suffering from depressive illness to deny the depressive mood, while admitting to somatic features (almost one-third of cases in our studies). Other patients are said to somatize depressed mood and exhibit what are termed "depressive equivalents," mimicking physical illness. Some authors have suggested that common factors may occasionally cause both depression and physical illness, and the occurrence of depression preceding the diagnosis of cancer is cited.

The association between depression and dementia has received some attention. After examining several hundreds of elderly patients in hospital and several thousand in the community, we formed the impression that the supposed difficulties of diagnosis are overemphasized. This is probably because of the considerable therapeutic importance of making the distinction and because those inexperienced in examining the elderly find it difficult to know how much of the clinical picture to impute to depression and how much to normal ageing, and because in clinical practice the examination is often conducted under adverse conditions in the patient's own home or on a busy hospital ward. A thorough clinical examination rarely leaves much doubt in most cases, but from time to time spectacular mistakes can be made, and so-called demented patients may appear quite normal at follow-up or to have developed obvious depression without organic features. Nor is the relationship always a simple one. Post-mortem studies by the Newcastle group showed that cases considered to be depression in life had higher plaque counts than would have been expected for normal ageing. More work is needed to resolve this relationship. The dexamethasone suppression test has proved a disappointing discriminator and CAT scanning has not proved as helpful as expected. Longitudinal studies are needed with improved clinical and radiological investigations on greater numbers of subjects.

Discussion

The prevalence of serious depression does not seem to vary much between different populations, and such variation that is reported is more likely to be due to different diagnostic criteria or the differing application of such criteria. However, the prevalence of serious depression is comparatively small and therefore will require larger studies with more tightly defined criteria, especially if division into bi- and unipolar groups is to be made.

The prevalence of minor forms of depression, which nevertheless cause considerable disability and suffering, does appear to vary between different locations. There is some evidence now to suggest that the prevalence of depression and life events are less in the rural than in the urban elderly, and that adverse social conditions in society do not necessarily lead to increased proportions of depression in this age group.

Depression in elderly community subjects and in those on general hospital wards continues to go untreated. Only 4% of our depressed community sample in Liverpool received treatment from their general practitioners specifically for depression while over 80% of the same subjects were receiving treatment for other medical conditions. It seems that depressive symptoms may be recognized, while not being considered worth treating.

Some depressive conditions appear to be truly reactive to a physical illness, improving when the latter improves, whilst others, more severe and perhaps fulfilling the criteria for major affective disorder, are precipitated by physical illness. It is known from the studies of Paykel et al. (1969) and Brown and Harris (1978) that adverse life events precede most kinds of depression, both the reactive or neurotic and the so-called endogenous or psychotic types. It would seem not unreasonable to suppose that physical illness acts like any other unpleasant life event associated with a loss of function, often permanent or semi-permanent. In the majority of individuals this is likely to result in a reactive illness such as dysthymia, or as we would prefer to call it, "morbid distress" (Copeland 1985), a term emphasizing its varied nature and continuum with normal behaviour. Clearly, a range of factors including social support and coping strategies are implicated. In those patients predisposed genetically, or by previous life experience (Brown et al. 1977), the depression may progress to major affective disorder, which in its turn may influence the prognosis of the physical condition. Whether conditions directly affecting the brain provoke another mechanism is not known.

Whether the apparent decline in the prevalence of depression in men in their 70s is due to a selective death of those predisposed to depression due to associated physical illness is also unknown. To solve many of the outstanding problems, longitudinal studies are necessary as well as further research on coping mechanisms (and why some patients with severe physical illness do not develop depression) and particularly on the influence of physical conditions (like endocrine disorders and drugs) on those brain areas controlling emotion. The entire intimate relationship between mind and body lies relatively unexplored.

References

American Psychiatric Association (1980) Diagnostic and statistical manual of mental disorders (DSM III). Washington, DC American Psychiatric Association

Blazer D (1982) The epidemiology of later life depression. J Geriatr Soc 30:587–592

Blazer D, Williams CD (1980) Epidemiology of dysphoria and depression in an elderly population. Am Psychiatry 137:439–444

Brown GW, Harris TO (1978) Social origins of depression. London, Tavistock

Brown GW, Harris TO, Copeland JRM (1977) Depression and loss. Br J Psychiatry 130:1–18

Bukberg J, Penman D, Holland JC (1984) Depression in hospitalized cancer patients. Psychosom Med 46(3):199–212

Connolly J (1976) Life events before myocardial infarction. J Human Stress 2:3–17

Cooper B, Schwarz R (1982) Psychiatric case-identification in an elderly urban population. Soc Psychiatry 17:43–52

Copeland JRM (1985) Depressive illness and morbid distress. Onset and development data examined against 5-year outcome. Br Psychiatry 146:297–307

Copeland JRM, Gurland BJ (1978) Evaluation of diagnostic methods: an international comparison. In: Issacs AD, Post F (eds) Studies in geriatric psychiatry. Wiley, Chichester, 189–209

Copeland JRM, Dewey ME, Griffiths-Jones HM (1986) A computerized psychiatric diagnostic system and case nomenclature for elderly subjects: GMS and AGECAT. Psycholog Med 16:89–99

Copeland JRM, Dewey ME, Wood N, Searle R, Davidson IA, McWilliam C (1987a) The range of mental illness amongst the elderly in the community: prevalence in Liverpool. Br J Psychiatry 150:815–823

Copeland JRM, Gurland BJ, Dewey ME, Kelleher MJ, Smith AMR, Davidson IA (1987b) Is there more dementia, depression and neurosis in New York? A comparative community study of the elderly in New York and London using the computer diagnosis AGECAT. Br J Psychiatry 151:446–473

Copeland JRM, Neal CD, Harrison MAM, McWilliam C, Dewey ME (1988) Is there more or less dementia and other mental illness amongst rural communities of elderly people? A pilot study using the GMS-AGECAT package (submitted for publication)

Feighner JP, Robins E, Guze SB, Woodruff RA, Winokur Q, Minoz R (1972) Diagnostic criteria for use in psychiatric research. Arch Gen Psychiatry 26:57–63

Gibson AC (1961) Psychosis occurring in the senium. J Men Sci 107:921

Gurland BJ, Copeland JRM, Kelleher MJ, Kuriansky J, Sharpe L, Dean L (1983) Mind and mood of aging: the mental health problems of the community elderly in New York and London. Haworth Press, New York London Croom Helm
Heine B, Sainsbury P (1970) Prolonged emotional disturbance and essential hypertension. Psychother Psychosom 18:341–348
Kay DWK, Bergmann K (1966) Physical disability and mental health in old age. J Psychosom Res 10:3–12
Kay DWK, Beamish R, Roth M (1964) Old age mental disorders in Newcastle on Tyne. Part 1. A study of prevalence. Br J Psychiatry 110:146–158
Kay DWK, Henderson AS, Scott R, Wilson J, Rickwood D, Grayson DA (1985) Dementia and depression among the elderly living in the Hobart community: the effect of the diagnostic criteria on the prevalence rates. Psycholog Med 15:771–788
Koranyi EK (1980) Somatic illness in psychiatric patients. Psychosomatics 21:887–891
Kramlinger KG, Swanso DW, Maruta T (1983) Are patients with chronic pain depressed? Am J Psychiatry 140:747–749
Lloyd GG (1977) Psychological reactions to physical illness. Br J Psychiatry 18:354–358
Mann AH, Graham N, Ashby D (1984) Psychiatric illness in residential homes for the elderly: a survey in one London Borough. Age Ageing 13:257–265
Moffic HS, Paykel ES (1973) Depression in medical inpatients. Br J Psychiatry 126:346–353
Morris PA (1962) A survey of 100 female senile admissions to a mental hospital. J Ment Sci 108:801
Murphy E (1983) The prognosis of depression in old age. Br J Psychiatry 142:111–119
Murphy E, Brown GW (1980) Life events, psychiatric disturbance, and physical illness. Br J Psychiatry 136:326–328
Nielsen J, Homma A, Biorn-Henriksen T (1977) Follow-up 15 years after a geronto-psychiatric prevalence study. Conditions concerning death, causes of death and life expectancy in relation to psychiatric diagnosis. J Gerontol 32:554–561
Paykel ES, Myers JK, Dienelt MN, Klerman GL, Lindenthal JI, Pepper MP (1969) Life events and depression: a controlled study. Arch Gen Psychiatry 21:753–760
Persson G (1980) Prevalence of mental disorders in a 70-year-old urban population. Acta Psychiatr Scand 62:119–139
Post F (1951) The outcome of mental breakdown in old age. Br Med J 1:436–448
Querido A (1959) Forecast and follow-up: an investigation into the physical, social and neutral factors determining the results of hospital treatment. Br J Prevent Soc Med 13:33–39
Rutter M (1963) Psychological factors in the short-term prognosis of physical disease. 1. Peptic ulcer. J Psychos Res 7:45–60
Roth M, Morrissey JD (1952) Problems in the diagnosis and classification of mental disorders of old age. J Ment Sci 98:66–88
Weissman MM, Myers JK (1980) Psychiatric disorders in a U.S. community. The application of research diagnostic criteria to a resurveyed community sample. Acta Psychiatr Scand 62:99–111

Comments: Mortality in Depressive Disorders; a 3-Year Prospective Follow-Up Study in Finland

J. LÖNNQVIST [1] and M. KOSKENVUO [2]

Introduction

Interaction between depression and somatic illness is a complex process with many feedback effects (Fig. 1). The adaptation process ranges from the specific etiological and background factors to the illness and further, through the subjective meanings of the illness and the coping strategies, to the outcome. The worst possible outcome is the death of a patient. The same kind of process of adaptation can be used for depression, too. The important question is whether and in which way these processes interact with each other. Components modify each other's functioning in a circular way, amplifying and/or weakening the main course of the process.

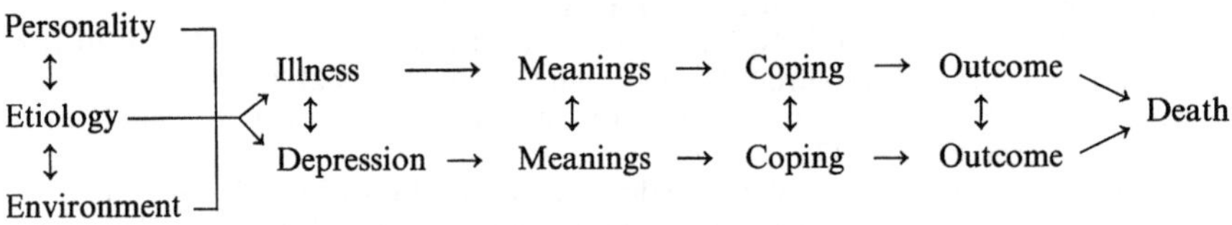

Fig. 1. Interaction between depression and somatic illness as a process model

Depression is a very basic, general, and complicated state of maladaptation. It would be very interesting to study why there are serious illnesses without depression and serious depressions without somatic consequences.

The Oxford record linkage study by Baldwin (1980) shows that among depressives there is an increased risk for ischemic heart disease, cerebrovascular diseases, and hypertension. Baldwin found also an elevated risk for pneumonia, bronchitis, pulmonary tuberculosis, asthma, hay fever, peptic ulcer, diabetes mellitus, thyreotoxicosis, and myxedema.

Just to summarize the literature on mortality in depressive disorders we can say that: (a) there is an increased mortality in affective disorders; (b) the mortality of the unipolar depressions is elevated as well as that of bipolar de-

[1] Department of Psychiatry and [2] Department of Public Health, University of Helsinki, SF-00290 Helsinki

Depressive Illness: Prediction of Course and Outcome
Edited by T. Helgason and R. J. Daly

pressions (Perris 1966; Tsuang et al. 1978); (c) the high mortality is not only due to the high rate of suicides but also due to physical diseases in general (Tsuang et al. 1978). The mortality in neurotic or milder depressions is not very well-known. Prospective and cause-specific studies are needed.

Material and Methods

All Finnish men aged 35–64 and treated in hospital for neurotic depression (300.4 in ICD-8) or affective psychoses (296 in ICD-8) in 1972 and alive at the end of 1972 were formed into two study cohorts. The number of patients with neurotic depression was 435 and with affective psychoses 348. The control cohort was formed in a similar way from three separate hospital cohorts: acute appendicitis ($n=1120$), haemorrhoids ($n=975$), and varicose veins ($n=1185$), altogether 3280 patients.

Computer files of hospital records and death certificates from the years 1972–1975 were used as a data base. The follow-up data were formed by linking the hospital records and death certificates for the years 1973, 1974, and 1975 to the cohorts under study. All deaths were checked manually for all cohorts in 5-year age groups. The expected number of deaths was calculated by each age group using the rates of the control cohort. Risk ratios were calculated from observed and expected figures and summed over all age groups.

Results

The overall mortality for depressive disorders was higher in all age groups compared to the control cohort during the 3-year follow-up period (Table 1).

The mortality was higher especially in younger age groups. The difference declined steadily by the age groups, but the ratio remained at two times higher

Table 1. Observed (O) and expected (E) deaths by age for neurotic depression (ND) and affective psychoses (AP) compared (O/E) to control cohort (CC) during the 3-year follow-up after hospitalization

Age (years)	ND ($n=435$)		AP ($n=348$)		ND+AP ($n=783$)		CC ($n=3280$)
	O	O/E	O	O/E	O	O/E	O
35–39	9	10.0	3	5.6	12	8.3	7
40–44	9	7.2	3	6.1	12	6.9	8
45–49	8	3.2	7	5.1	15	3.8	15
50–54	4	1.7	11	4.0	15	3.0	18
55–59	5	2.4	5	1.9	10	2.1	20
60–64	3	1.4	9	2.2	12	2.0	26

after 55 years old. There were no significant differences between neurotic depression and affective psychoses in total mortality, yet the ratio was higher for neurotic depression, between 35–44 years.

For natural causes of death the risk ratio was significantly higher both in neurotic depression (2.5) and in affective psychoses (2.3), compared with the control cohort during the 3-year follow-up period (Table 2).

The proportion of natural deaths was 5.3% in neurotic depression, 6.6% in affective psychoses, and 2.2% in the control group.

The ischemic heart disease mortality risk ratios were for neurotic depression 2.3 and for affective psychoses 1.8 (Table 3).

Ischemic heart disease was the cause of death in 1.8% for neurotic depression and in 2.0% for affective psychoses.

The specific causes of natural deaths for all neurotic depressions ($n=435$) were as follows: ischemic heart disease 8, cerebral embolus 2, arteriosclerosis 1, lung embolus 1, pneumonia 1, emphysema 1, diabetes 1, cirrhosis 1, alcoholism 1, pulmonary carcinoma 4 and ventricular carcinoma 2.

The risk of violent death for depressive patients is presented in Table 4. The risk ratio for neurotic depression was 5.0 and for affective psychoses 5.9.

The risk of suicide was very high both for neurotic depression (30.2) and for affective psychoses (33.0). The risk ratio during the 1st follow-up year for neurotic depression was as high as 72.5 and for affective psychoses 53.3 (Table 5).

The proportions of natural deaths, suicides, and other violent deaths in all three cohorts are presented in Table 6. Natural deaths were dominating in the control group and suicides in the cohort of affective psychoses.

Table 2. Mortality risk ratios for natural causes of deaths in neurotic depression (ND), affective psychoses (AP), and control cohort (CC) during the 3-year follow-up

Cohort	Size	Natural deaths		Risk ratio
	(*n*)	(*n*)	(%)	
ND	435	23	5.3	2.7
AP	348	23	6.6	2.6
CC	3280	72	2.2	1.0

Table 3. Observed (O) and expected (E) number of deaths for ischemic heart diseases (IHD) and cerebrovascular diseases (CVD) in neurotic depression (ND) and in affective psychoses (AP) compared (O/E) to the control cohort (CC) during the 3-year follow-up period

Cause of death	ND			AP			CC
	O	E	O/E	O	E	O/E	O
IHD	8	3.5	2.3	7	3.9	1.9	29
CVD	2	0.9	2.4	4	0.9	4.4	7

Table 4. The risk of violent deaths of depressive patients during the 3-year follow-up period

Cohort	Size	Violent deaths	Risk ratio
Neurotic depression	435	15	5.0
Affective psychoses	348	15	5.9
Control cohort	3280	22	1.0

Table 5. The risk of suicide of depressive patients during the 3-year follow-up period

Cohort	Size	Suicides	Risk ratios	
			1973	1973–1975
Neurotic depression	435	10	72.5	30.2
Affective psychoses	348	13	53.3	33.0
Control cohort	3280	4	1.0	1.0

Table 6. Proportion (%) of natural deaths (ND), suicides (S), and other violent deaths (OVD) of the depressive patients during the 3-year follow-up period

Cohort	ND	S	OVD
Neurotic depression	61.5	25.6	12.8
Affective psychoses	60.5	34.2	5.3
Control cohort	76.6	4.2	19.1

Concluding Remarks

In our 3-year prospective follow-up study on all Finnish men aged 35–64 treated in hospital in 1972 for neurotic depression or for affective psychoses, we could confirm the basic findings of Baldwin (1980). There is an increased risk for natural causes of death in neurotic depression and in affective psychoses.

We do not know which are the linking mechanisms behind these correlations. It seems that there are many and that it is possible to study them on different levels of human systems. One useful level is human behaviour, for example, smoking as risk behaviour. Another level to study connections between depression and mortality is an intrapsychic use of defence mechanisms, for example, excessive use of denial, splitting, and projective and introjective mechanisms. We can study depression in biological systems, too. However, what we need is integrating models which could explain the dynamics between these various kinds of subsystems. We could begin with intensive and prospective case studies.

In addition, there are very high suicide risks for neurotic depression and for affective psychoses. It is important to note, that the risk of suicide for so-called neurotic depressions, if treated in hospital, is as high as that for affective psychoses. Actually it is higher during the first follow-up year. It seems that we have so-called neurotic depressions, which, when treated in hospital, have poor outcome.

Outcome as measured by mortality does not seem to validate the concepts of neurotic and affective psychoses as separate entities.

References

Baldwin JA (1980) Schizophrenia and physical disease: a preliminary analysis of data from the Oxford Record Linkage Study. In: Hemmings G (ed) The biochemistry of schizophrenia and addiction. MTP Press, Lancaster, pp 297–318

Perris C (1966) A study of bipolar (manic-depressive) and unipolar recurrent affective psychoses. Acta Psychiatr Scand 42 (Suppl 194)

Tsuang MT, Woolson RF (1978) Excess mortality in schizophrenia and affective disorders: do suicides and accidental deaths solely account for this excess? Arch Gen Psychiatry 35:1181–1185

Personality as a Mediating Variable in the Pathogenesis of Mood Disorders: Implications for Theory, Research, and Prevention *

H. S. AKISKAL

Introduction

It is widely believed that affective episodes arise from predisposing personality attributes. This position was most directly articulated by Kretschmer (1936), who believed that "the endogenous psychoses are nothing but accentuation of normal types of temperament." While Kretschmer, as a faithful follower of the Kraepelinian tenets (1921), emphasized constitutionally determined temperamental contributions, much current theorizing has focused on learned characterologic attributes, believed to be the legacy of developmental vicissitudes (Chodoff 1972). Ideally, the study of personality in a given patient should precede the first affective episode as affective states may bias or even mask the patient's personality profile. Even during euthymic periods, personality structure is altered by the illness episodes or the treatments provided for them. For these reasons, very few studies have succeeded in prospectively assessing the contribution of personality to mood disorders. However, despite the methodologic barriers, many interesting findings on the relevance of enduring personality characteristics to mood disorders have been recently reported.

In this paper I will develop the thesis that personality represents the intermediary stage between remote (e.g., hereditary and developmental) and proximate (e.g., precipitating) causative factors in the origin of full-blown mood disorders. According to this model (Fig. 1), depressive and manic episodes arise from the matrix of premorbid personality characteristics which tend to persist when episodes subside. Short-term interpersonal maladjustments which result from the interaction of premorbid personality, symptoms of the episode, and the social environment often crystallize into permanent postaffective personality maladjustments, especially in recurrent mood disorders. These maladjustments, in turn, provide fertile ground for the development of subsequent episodes and, in the worst possible case, contribute to suicidal outcome.

In discussing the available literature bearing on these issues, I will argue that in predicting the outcome of mood disorders (recurrence, bipolar switches, scholastic, vocational or conjugal failure, or suicide), it is essential

Section of Affective Disorders, University of Tennessee, Memphis, TN 38163, USA

* Parts of this chapter previously appeared in Akiskal H (1984), Characterologic manifestations of affective disorders: toward a new conceptualization (Integr Psychiatry 2:83–88) and are reproduced here by permission of Elsevier Science Publishing Co., New York

Depressive Illness: Prediction of Course and Outcome
Edited by T. Helgason and R. J. Daly

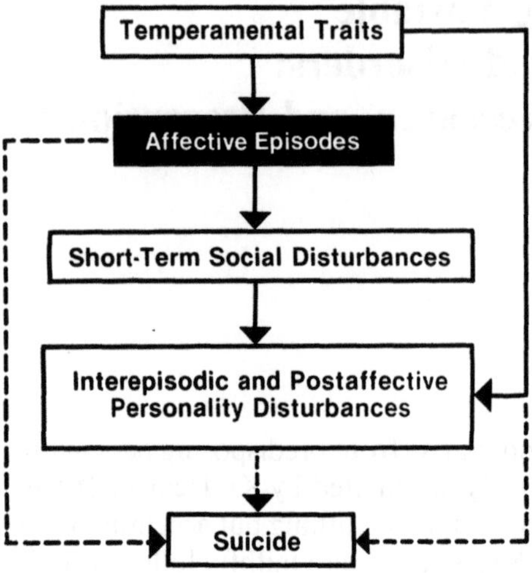

Fig. 1. Schematic representation of the relationship between personality, episodes, and outcome in recurrent mood disorders

to take the intermorbid personality into consideration. Finally, I will present some thoughts on how such a model can contribute to efforts designed to prevent the more serious outcome in mood disorders. Throughout this review I will highlight recent empirical findings; for a fuller account of the theoretical position within which these findings are reviewed, the reader is referred to previous publications (Akiskal 1984, 1985, 1987a; Akiskal and Mckinney 1975; Akiskal et al. 1983a).

Personality as a Subaffective Expression of Mood Disorders

Both psychoanalytic and descriptive biologic approaches to mental disorders have recognized the importance of genetic factors. In the Freudian conceptualization (1959), the term genetic denotes developmental unfolding of constitution into characterologic constellations that predispose to adult psychopathology; thus, "double fixation" at oral and anal stages is believed to cause the excessive interpersonal dependency and rigid obsessionalism that predispose to morbid oscillations of mood (Abraham 1960). By contrast, in the Kraepelinian schema (1921), developed to its fullest in the work of Kretschmer (1936) and Lange (1928) the hereditary potential finds expression in a spectrum of disorders ranging from the affective temperaments to the affective psychoses. Here, the milder oscillations of mood represented by the temperaments serve as the background from which the more severe forms of the illness arise. While the relative emphasis accorded to early experience vs heredity differs in these formulations, they seem to converge in considering personality disturbances as the *fundamental* pathology from which the more florid symptomatic phases of the illness arise. Thus, personality could represent as much an expression of the affective pathology as the more classic symptomatic episodes of the illness. Such a conceptualization would posit that many of the personality disturbances associated with mood disorders represent subaffective (i.e., attenuated) expressions of these disorders (Akiskal 1984).

The Cyclothymic Temperament

When the University of Tennessee Mood Clinic was established in the mid-1970s, we were confronted with a large number of patients who were moody, impulsive, erratic, and volatile, but who did not meet the duration and syndromal criteria for manic-depressive illness (Akiskal et al. 1977, 1979). They presented to our clinic primarily because of repeated romantic or conjugal failure in the context of the following social and interpersonal disturbances:

- Episodic promiscuity
- Geographic instability (i.e., history of repeated changes of city or residence)
- Dilettantism in academic and professional pursuits
- Uneven work record
- Brief affiliations with various eschatological cults, typically followed by disillusionment within a short period of time
- Episodic pattern of substance and alcohol abuse, alternating between sedatives and stimulants

These disturbances explain why most of these patients had received personality labels such as passive-aggressive, histrionic, borderline, or antisocial. Only after in-depth phenomenologic study and prospective follow-up did it become clear that their personality maladjustments reflected underlying phasic affective dysregulation. The temperamental disturbances that characterized these cyclothymic probands were more in the spheres of psychomotor functioning and behavior than mood per se. They alternated between short cycles (typically lasting a few days) of drive and lethargy; euthymic periods were relatively uncommon. Decreased need for sleep was followed by slothful hypersomnolence, creative spurts by intellectual aridity, arrogant and naive overconfidence by sudden and unexplained lowering of self-esteem, hedonistic pursuits by apathetic withdrawal, and people-seeking by self-isolation; in general, passionate involvement in things gave way to a sudden loss of joie de vivre. These patients often used terms like "high" and "low" in describing their humor, which alternated between irritable, often nervous moods and emotional quietude, or rapidly went from explosive angry outbursts to guilty self-recriminations. Characteristically, these changes were sudden, with little discernible relationship to interpersonal or family pressures. If anything, these patients' personal crises in the form of object losses often appeared to result from their unpredictability. In support of this suggestion are data from a recent study

(Klein et al. 1985) showing that the cyclothymic offspring of bipolar patients have far greater disruption in their social lives than their noncyclothymic siblings.

The affective basis of the "characterologic" disturbances reviewed above was validated by the significant excess of full-blown depressive and hypomanic/manic episodes compared with nonaffective personality disordered controls during prospective observation; as many as one-third of these episodes were mobilized by tricyclic antidepressants. Further, the family histories of these patients were essentially identical to those of controls with classic manic-depressive illness.

These findings document that attenuated cyclothymic forms of bipolar illness do exist in the outpatient setting and that the most visible pathology in this group of patients is manifested in a tempestuous lifestyle that creates interpersonal havoc.

The Hyperthymic Temperament

Life-long hypomanic adjustment is so adaptive in work- and activity-oriented societies that it is rarely considered to represent a form of psychopathology. The drive and self-assured entrepreneurial attitude characteristic of hypomanic individuals often places them in leadership roles where their less-desirable uninhibited and meddlesome traits are tolerated. Although their intensity tends to drive others away, their exuberance and people-seeking behavior are counterbalancing assets. Impaired judgment in social, sexual, and financial spheres may hurt their loved ones and irritate associates; lack of insight and a hypertrophied sense of denial prevents them from seeking psychiatric help even when these behaviors lead to personal disasters. They present to psychiatric settings only when the development of explosive mania or paralyzing depression forces their lovel ones to take action on their behalf.

It is of theoretical significance that the extroverted, ambitious, and driven person with an inordinate capacity for work – Sjöbring's "substable" profile for the bipolar personality (Nyman 1956) – overlaps considerably with the duty-bound work-addicted "anancastic" (compulsive) personality of the Anglo-Saxon literature (American Psychiatric Association 1980). The "typus melancholicus" described by Tellenbach (1980) as the characterologic constellation predisposed to melancholic episodes also overlaps to some extent with the hyperthymic adjustment described above. Such individuals are extremely dedicated to work and find little time for leisure; their "dynamism," however, appears artificial, and is usually considered an overcompensated "defense" against depressive tendencies.

These affinities between hypomanic and melancholic personality types find further support in sleep studies. In the Sleep Disorders Center affiliated with our Mood Clinic, 12 work-addicted individuals with hyperthymic personality have been observed during the past decade (Akiskal 1984). Most presented with the chief complaint of insomnia; nearly all were highly energetic and successful people in leadership positions or in lucrative businesses who, over the years, had typically needed only 4–5 h of sleep nightly. However, they had been intermittently bothered by "nervous energy" and inability to sleep; now, in late middle age, alcohol – after being effective for many years – no longer put them to sleep. After many years of exceptional physical fitness, they were concerned about their failing physiology, reflected in sleep difficulty. These patients vigorously denied depressive and other psychiatric symptoms, and had extremely low Beck depression and MMPI scores. Yet their REM latencies during sleep polysommographic study were as short as those of primary depressives.

Data generated in our sleep laboratory (Akiskal 1983a) indicate that significant shortening of this neurophysiologic marker of primary depressive illness may represent a trait abnormality that is present during interepisodic as well as episodic phases of illness. Abnormally shortened REM latency, while not unexpected in depressive personality, is somewhat unexpected in hypomanic personality. However, the driven work habits of hypomanic individuals suggest that their adjustment is brittle and may have an underlying depressive component.

To recapitulate, although the personality expressions of a hyperthymic mode of existence are often represented in highly adaptive extroverted traits and an enormous capacity for work, they appear to be superimposed on unstable affective adjustment. This may explain the liability of the hyperthymic temperament to both major depressive and manic breakdowns.

The Dysthymic Temperament

Low-grade chronic depressive manifestations occur in the setting of a variety of psychopathologic conditions. For instance, some individuals develop chronic pessimism, low self-confidence, self-critical attitudes, passivity, and interpersonal dependency *following* well-defined depressive episodes from which they do not recover completely. Such sequelae are best described as "post-depressive personality" (Cassano et al. 1983). Still others develop chronic depressive attitudes in the setting of such conditions as agoraphobia, obsessive-compulsive disorder, anorexia nervosa, ego-dystonic homosexuality, and so on. In both of these cases, the depressive personality characteristics are best conceptualized as complications of, or inadequate recovery from, major psychiatric disorders (Akiskal 1983b).

Of greater interest to our discussion of personality as a subaffective expression of mood disorder are patients who report they have "always" (at least since their teens) had depressive tendencies. In clinical parlance, such individuals are often considered "characterologic depressives" (Akiskal et al. 1980; Rosenthal et al. 1981). This term is apt inasmuch as it connotes the difficulty in separating the depressive elements from the character structure. Self-hatred, habitual gloom, and self-denigration are so deeply ingrained in these individuals that they appear to be part of the personality structure. These charactero-logically expressed affective disturbances represent a heterogeneous group of patients generally considered resistant to most treatment modalities. The disappointing results with pharmacotherapy can perhaps be explained by failure to address these patients' lack of social adroitness; similarly, psychotherapy always seems impotent in reversing the temperamentally based inertia characteristic of such patients.

In a University of Tennessee study (Akiskal et al. 1980) of characterologic depressives, two distinct groups were identified on the basis of response to behavioral modalities like social skills training with a vigorous trial of several tricyclic antidepressants and/or lithium carbonate. Those who respond to such combined treatment were hypothesized to represent an attenuated or a *subaffective* dysthymic disorder in view of family history (often bipolar in nature), superimposed major depressive episodes, and hypomanic responses to antidepressant drugs. It is noteworthy that even when examined in their habitual or trait condition - i.e., when not in a definable depressive episode – these patients had the shortened REM latency characteristic of primary depressive states. By contrast, the nonresponsive group had the features of a primary charactero-logic disorder (hysteroid-antisocial features, normal REM latency, familial alcoholism, familial assortative mating, and high rates of developmental object loss) and was classified as having a character-spectrum disorder.

The findings reviewed above support the notion that some individuals with introverted, obsessoid, and masochistic features, who are habitually brooding, guilt-ridden, gloomy, pessimistic, self-denigrating, anhedonic, and tend to oversleep are suffering from a clinically attenuated but lifelong form of melancholia. These features are remarkably reminiscent of Schneider's description (1958) of the depressive psychopath. Careful evaluation of their lethargy often reveals psychomotor inertia, which is particularly pronounced in the morning hours. Furthermore, although habitually introverted, these individuals may, for brief periods of time, appear extroverted and driven. These extroverted tendencies reach the threshold of clinical hypomania only when the patient is treated with tricyclic antidepressants. Table 1 compares the respective rates of

Table 1. Affective episodes (in percentages) in affective temperaments and nonaffective personality disorder controls during 1–4 years prospective observation. (From Akiskal et al. 1977, 1980)[a]

	Cyclothymic ($n=46$)	Subaffective dysthymic ($n=20$)	Controls ($n=50$)
Major depression	24	55	4
Hypomanic/mania (spontaneous)	22	0	0
Tricyclic-hypomania	35	33	0

[a] Experimental groups significantly higher than controls ($p<0.02$).

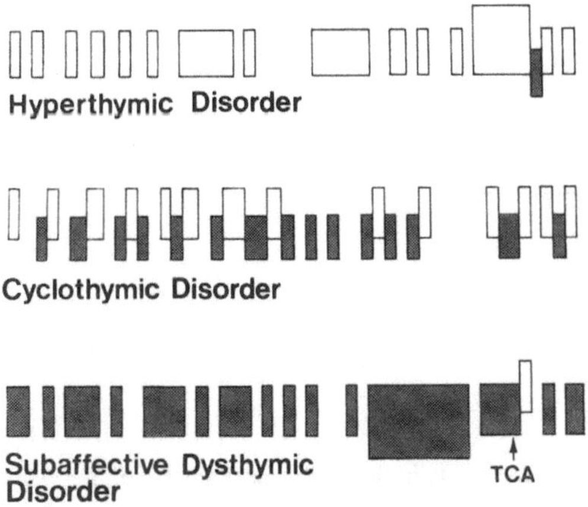

Fig. 2. Schematic representation of the three affective temperaments. *White rectanglas* represent hypomanic periods and *grey ones,* depressive

major depressive, spontaneous hypomanic or manic, and tricyclic-mobilized hypomanic episodes in subaffective dysthymic subjects with those of cyclothymic and nonaffective personality disorder controls. Except for spontaneous hypomania, these rates are comparable in dysthymics and cyclothymics and elevated from those of nonaffective personality controls. Such data suggest that the subaffective dysthymic temperament as defined by us appears to be a less penetrant form of cyclothymic disorder (Fig. 2), representing a subtle expression of central affective dysregulation that is manifest predominantly in phasic "minidepressions" (Akiskal 1983 b).

Individuals with dysthymic temperament are unable to enjoy leisure and tend to be extremely dedicated to work that requires selfless devotion and much attention to detail. However, this stable adjustment in the vocational sphere is not paralleled in social adjustment (DeLisio et al. 1987). The sombre personalities and intense attachment needs of these individuals may drive others away. Such interpersonal losses then cause them to sink into lower depths of black humor. Recent prospective studies have indeed shown that depressive personalities are at considerable risk of developing major depressive breakdowns, leading to the "double depressive" pattern, i.e., major depressive episodes superimposed on low-grade depressions (Keller and Shapiro 1982).

Theoretical and Research Implications

A Multicausal Etiological Scheme

The full exposition of the multicausal scheme whereby genetic and developmental factors interact in giving rise to personality disturbances has been re-

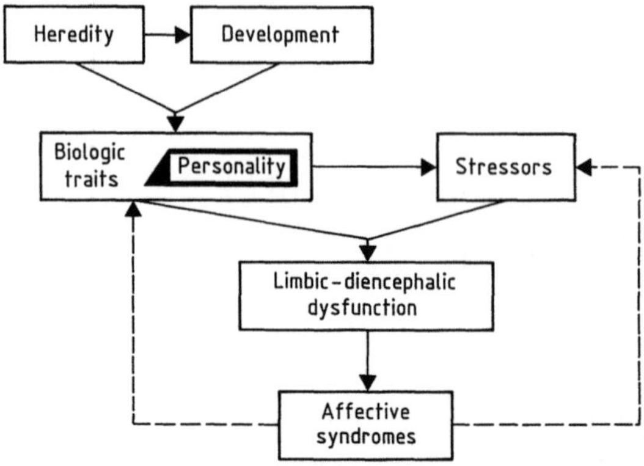

Fig. 3. The hypothesized mediating role of personality in the multicausal scheme of mood disorders

viewed elsewhere (Akiskal 1985; Akiskal and McKinney 1975; Akiskal et al. 1983a). In this scheme, affective personalities are conceived as intermediary between remote and proximate etiologic factors, on the one hand, and the biologic and clinical manifestations of the mood disorders, on the other (Fig. 3). The impact of proximate stressors on the vulnerable limbic-diencephalic substrates of the organism and the ultimate translation of such vulnerability into the overt clinical picture of the affective syndromes have also been elaborated in previous work (Akiskal and McKinney 1975). What I have described here are recent findings on the personality attributes and associated sleep neurophysiologic traits commonly observed in the premorbid and intermorbid phase of mood disorders. At an observable level, these attributes and traits are manifested in hyperthymic, cyclothymic, dysthymic, and related behavioral patterns. These patterns are shaped by and interact with the risk factors (Akiskal 1985, 1987a, b) diagrammed in Fig. 3, and detailed below, in giving rise to overt clinical episodes of mood disorder:

- Positive family history for mood disorder, especially "loaded" pedigrees in three consecutive generations
- Exposure to depressed patients during childhood and/or early breaks in attachment bonds without adequate parenting substrates
- Disabling physical illnesses and/or drug treatment of such, especially those affecting the central nervous system
- Use of steroid contraceptives
- Subclinical hypothyroidism
- Life events – especially losses – in the setting of minimal supportive social ties

Additional risk factors (Akiskal 1985, 1987a, b) particularly relevant for bipolar episodes include:

- Treatment with or abuse of catecholaminergic drugs
- Sleep deprivation

- The premenstrual phase
- The postpartum period
- Seasonal photoperiodic changes

Personality as a Mediating Variable in Affective Recurrences

The findings reviewed here have been presented within the framework of the classical view that certain temperamental disorders – the dysthymic, the hyperthymic, and the cyclothymic – are the precursors of the more serious and recurrent affective episodes. Recent data from three different sources suggest that bipolar disorder may be inherited in the form of these temperaments: (a) the "discordant" member in a monozygotic pair in about one-third of cases exhibits one of these temperamental disturbances (Bertelsen et al. 1977); (b) the preponderance of such disturbances in the teenage as well as prepubertal offspring of bipolars (Akiskal et al. 1985); and (c) similar rates of bipolar family history in all affective temperaments when compared with seriously ill hospitalized bipolars (Akiskal 1984). It would therefore appear that in these temperaments, the genetic potential for affective episodes is subclinically active at all times and easily triggered by environmental challenge. It is interesting that all three temperaments are at risk for depressive episodes, and hypomania is augmented by exposure to tricyclic antidepressants.

Recent Italian work by Kukopulus et al. (1980) suggests that tricyclic antidepressants may actually *accelerate* the inherent cyclicity of mood disorders in hyperthymic and cyclothymic individuals. Our findings (Akiskal et al. 1985) on the 3- to 4-year prospective course in the juvenile offspring and sibs of adult bipolars (Table 2) support this view; juvenile subjects with depressive onsets (and treated largely with tricyclic antidepressants) had a significantly higher rate of recurrence – including rapid-cycling – compared with those with hypomanic or manic onsets (and treated with lithium carbonate).

It can be concluded that certain affective personalities are at high risk for developing depressive states under conditions of environmental challenge;

Table 2. Three-year outcome (in percentages) of depressive vs manic and mixed onsets in juvenile offspring or sibs of bipolars. (Summarized from Akiskal 1985)[a]

	Depressive onsets ($n=24$)	Manic and mixed onsets ($n=11$)
Depressive	42	18
Hypomanic and mixed	30	18
Both	0	18
Rapid-cycling	8	0
Total with recurrence	80	54

[a] Recurrence in depressive onsets significantly greater than in manic and mixed onsets ($p=0.01$, two-tailed).

such stressors may also bring about hypomanic or manic states which can be facilitated by antidepressant challenges. Thus, it appears that one mechanism whereby genetic factors may produce episodes is via the instability of the affective temperaments. This viewpoint is strengthened by the recent demonstration of shortened REM latency in individuals with dysthymic and hyperthymic temperaments, very much like the findings in those experiencing major full-blown depressions. This sleep neurophysiologic abnormality seems to behave like a trait marker of vulnerability and is not merely a nonspecific stress reaction or a correlate of anxiety (Akiskal et al. 1984). Overall, the sleep findings in affective temperaments suggest that neurophysiologic abnormalities precede full-blown affective episodes.

Temperamental contributions appear to have greater relevance in the recurrent and cyclic forms of mood disorder (Akiskal 1984; Akistal et al. 1983 a). In the noncyclic forms of mood disorder, dependency and obsessionalism have long been hypothesized as predisposing factors (Chodoff 1972). More recent formulations have focused on cognitive-behavioral factors (Kovacs and Beck 1978; Lewinsohn 1974). However, these hypotheses have been developed through retrospective reconstruction of the premorbid characteristics of already depressed subjects. Other limitations include the use of small clinical populations, failure to take the heterogeneity of mood disorders into consideration, lack of reliable personality measures, and, most seriously, a tendency to confuse state and trait. A recent study (Hirschfield et al. 1983), which – except for its retrospective nature – was methodically superior to earlier attempts, reported that introversion, lack of social adroitness, and dependency are the major attributes of recovered depressives. These findings are more consistent with behavioral formulations and suggest the existence of enduring, measurable deficits in social skills. Prospective studies are now needed to clarify definitively the characterologic contributions in mood disorders.

In the absence of data from carefully designed prospective studies, clinical experience suggests mechanisms whereby the postulated characterologic disturbances contribute to major affective episodes. Individuals who are introverted and lack social adroitness do not possess an adequate behavioral repertoire for eliciting rewarding interactions. In particular, they may lack the requisite skills to develop and maintain the supportive relationships that are widely believed to provide a buffer against the depressogenic impact of aversive life situations. Passive-dependent individuals can easily exhaust the tolerance of their spouses or lovers and thereby prepare the ground for marital or romantic failures. In other words, they may contribute to the very life situations that bring about their depressive breakdowns. Once they become depressed, their dependency needs grow, increasing the likelihood of alienating the supportive individuals in their lives. The relationship between personality and mood disorder, however, is not always etiologic (Akiskal et al. 1983 a). Personality may favor the appearance of certain *symptoms* if and when an affective episode occurs; it may modify the apparent severity of the depressive state; and, in many instances, the characteristics described above *result* from recurrently incapacitating episodes of illness.

Taking mania as a paradigm (Akiskal 1983 c) one can argue that the behaviors of hyperthymic and cyclothymic personality give rise to the very situations that favor the full expression of the illness. These include (a) object losses resulting from alienation of loved ones or bringing about other personal crises; (b) sleep deprivation associated with a frantic social life or staying awake for worthy or unworthy pursuits; (c) childbirth (many are impulsively hypersexual); (d) treatment with tricyclic antidepressants (prescribed for retarded depression); and (e) abuse of psychedelics or stimulant drugs to further augment their work efficiency or excitement. It would therefore appear that the life course of a bipolar mood disorder has a momentum that, over time, augments the intensity of premorbid and intermorbid temperamental disturbances in the direction of greater cyclicity. Conceptualizing the origin of affective illness and its recurrences along the lines presented here should help to identify individuals predisposed to major affective breakdowns as well as delineating risk periods that should be taken into consideration in designing prevention efforts (Akiskal 1987 b).

Implications for Attenuating Long-Term Course

Many, although not all, of the findings reviewed in this article have been derived from retrospective or cross-sectional studies that have attempted to correlate a given clinical picture with various predictors. The time has now come to test these findings in prospective prevention research – just as is being done in studying hypertension and coronary artery disease. I will outline some of the possibilities of such preventive efforts. A fuller account can be found in a report prepared for a recent National Institute of Mental Health symposium (Akiskal 1987 b).

Primary Prevention

At least 10% of the population is estimated to be at risk of a clinically significant affective episode (Helgason 1979). Positive family history – especially when loaded – ist the most unambiguous major risk factor for recurrent mood disorders (Akiskal 1985, 1986). The risk for offspring is highest when both parents are ill. The risk is also high for the monzygotic co-twin of an affected individual; many of those co-twins will exhibit cyclothymic or dysthymic tendencies. Given the potential adverse effects of chronic lithium use, it would not be advisable to prescribe prophylactic lithium indiscriminately to this at-risk group. However, in the case of a cyclothymic woman with a loaded bipolar family history, it would be logical to prescribe lithium for a few months immediately postpartum. Also, cyclothymic and hyperthymic members of bipolar families should be educated to avoid sleep deprivation and catecholaminergic drugs – e.g., caffeine, other CNS stimulants, antidepressants, and other adrenergic vasoconstrictive and bronchodilator medications. Education of primary care physicians on the risks of prescribing certain depressant drugs (e.g., steroid contraceptives, antihypertensives) to patients with a positive family history may be the major practical approach to a primary prevention strategy at this stage of our knowledge.

Secondary Prevention

Here the aim is to prevent affective recurrences. The most logical group to focus on would be those who are at risk by virtue of family history and who have developed a mild (first) episode. Avoiding the prescription of depressant drugs is even more important for an individual who has already experienced an episode. Social skills training and vocational counselling might be beneficial for dysthymic and related personalities who seem to achieve optimum psychobiologic homeostasis if engaged in jobs that best fit their temperamental propensities. For instance, dysthymic individuals may do best in jobs that require loyalty, attention to detail, and self-sacrifice (e.g., civil service, secretarial jobs, bookkeeping, etc.). No data are available on whether traditional psychodynamic or more recent psychotherapeutic approaches such as cognitive therapy can prevent affective recurrences. Given that it is virtually impossible to reduce exposure to stressful life circumstances, however, improving coping mechanisms conceivably could reduce the perceived aversiveness of life events. Alternatively, one could introduce "protective" factors – such as social support – during stressful times to buffer the impact of stressors on individuals at risk. However, the value of such interventions in reducing affective recurrences is probably limited. This may in part be due to the fact that stressful events and the loss of social support are often by-products of the intermorbid temperament, which is not easily modifiable by psychotherapy.

With currently available techniques, prevention of major recurrences can best be accomplished with lithium carbonate. Lithium may be beneficial not only because it obviates the disruptive influence of illness episodes, but also because there is some attenuation of interepisodic temperamental instability. Considerable psychotherapeutic effort is obviously necessary to ensure compliance with medication regimens.

Recent research (Akiskal 1982) indicates that the group at greatest risk for the switch from unipolar to bipolar illness are young (<25 years), acutely ill, hypersomnic-retarded, often psychotic depressives with loaded (three generations) bipolar familial history. Even with a first episode, such patients should be treated with electroconvulsive therapy or lithium carbonate. Other measures include: (a) instructing the patient to avoid the use of stimulant drugs; (b) educating the patient about the risks of sleep deprivation and treating insomnia promptly with a short-term course of a sedating phenothiazine; and (c) avoiding the prescription of catecholaminergic heterocyclic antidepressants or limiting their use to small doses over short periods. In patients whose illness has a seasonal pattern, lithium prophylaxis limited to vulnerable periods (e.g., September through May) can be justified on clinical grounds. In such patients, depression can also be reduced by exposure to bright white light at home during periods of increased risk, as determined by past history of periodicity. However, this strategy carries the risk of inducing hypomania.

Tertiary Prevention

The effort here is to minimize or avert complications, which include substance abuse, social (especially marital) dysfunction, symptomatic chronicity, and suicide.

With respect to substance abuse, continuing and increased efforts to educate primary care physicians about the risks of sedative hypnotics are essential. The residual symptoms of affective episodes – which may linger for many months – should be vigorously treated with thymoleptic agents. Anxiolytic and hypnotic agents are rarely indicated; if prescribed, their use should not extend beyond a few weeks. Unfortunately, relatively little can be done to reduce abuse of ethanol, which patients tend to use to treat their insomnia.

Social complications can best be prevented by vigorous chemotherapy for acute episodes, combined with interpersonal psychotherapy. In dealing with symptomatic chronicity (Akiskal 1982), continued thymoleptic treatment, avoidance of depressant medical drugs, and supportive social measures are extremely important. Rates of chronic depression are especially high among individuals with severe, disabling, and long-lasting medical illness. This group should constitute a priority in prevention efforts. Group therapy and education of families or significant others could enhance these supportive social measures.

Since two-thirds of complete suicides are in individuals with mood disorders, vigorous treatment of these disorders should lead to decreases in suicide rates. However, despite promising data from mood disorders clinics (Khuri and Akiskal 1983), this ideal has not been reached at a community or national level. Murphy's data (1975) suggest that many primary care physicians not only underdiagnose mood disorders, but provide patients with lethal supplies of sedative drugs given as hypnotic agents.

It would appear that no significant prevention of suicidal behavior can occur untill all physicians are educated in the diagnosis and appropriate management of mood disorders. However, recent developments in the management of coma resulting from overdose of various psychoactive drugs may have reduced the actual mortality of suicide attempts. An increasing number of suicide victims – at least in the United States of America – are using violent methods such as firearms, so gun control legislation (though unlikely to be passed in the near future) might eventually prove useful in reducing suicidal mortality (Boyd 1983). Many victims of suicide by violent methods have evidence of strong elements of impulsivity and hostility in their personality structure (Clayton 1985). Such attributes, characteristically seen in the premorbid and intermorbid temperaments of those with recurrent mood disorders, are generally believed to be correlates of central serotonergic underfunction. These considerations are of interest in view of the recent claim by Åsberg et al. (1983) that lowered cerebrospinal fluid levels of 5-hydroxy-indoleacetic acid – an index of brain serotonin turnover – are predictive of violent suicidal acts, and raise the provocative (but hitherto unattained) possibility of treating such individuals with thymoleptic agents that tend to normalize central serotonergic homeostasis (e.g., lithium carbonate, trazodone, fluoxetine).

Since Kraepelin's time, it has been known that improvement in psychomotor retardation precedes mood uplifting and removes the inertia that may have prevented the patient's acting on suicidal urges. Therefore, in all suicide prevention efforts, it is obviously necessary not only to treat the mood disorder vigorously, but also to institute individualized psychotherapy, emphasizing round-the-clock vigilance or availability of help from the clinician and significant others. It is also necessary in hospitalized patients to avoid early discharge – an effort contrary to current third-party payment policies.

In summary, what is needed in prevention efforts is to go beyond the rhetoric of social psychiatry and institute programs that are soundly based on clinical research findings. Such efforts may not only lead to better prediction of the course of mood disorders, but hopefully to its attenuation in the foreseeable future.

References

Abraham K (1960) Notes on the psychoanalytic investigation and treatment of manic-depressive insanity and allied conditions. In: Selected papers on psychoanalysis. Basic Books, New York, pp 137–156

Akiskal HS (1982) Factors associated with incomplete recovery in primary depressive illness. J Clin Psychiatry 43:266–271

Akiskal HS (1983a) Diagnosis and classification of affective disorders: new insights from clinical and laboratory approaches. Psychiatr Dev 1:123–160

Akiskal HS (1983b) Dysthymic disorder: psychopathology of proposed chronic depressive subtypes. Am J Psychiatry 140:11–20

Akiskal HS (1983c) The bipolar spectrum: new concepts in classification and diagnosis. In: Grinspoon L (ed) Psychiatry update: the American Psychiatric Association annual review, vol 2. American Psychiatric Press, Washington, D.C., pp 271–292

Akiskal HS (1984) Characterologic manifestations of affective disorders: toward a new conceptualization. Integr Psychiatry 2:83–88

Akiskal HS (1985) Interaction of biologic and psychologic factors in the origin of depressive disorders. Acta Psychiatr Scand 71:131–139

Akiskal HS (1986) A developmental perspective on recurrent mood disorders: a review of studies in man. Psychopharmacol Bull 22:579–586

Akiskal HS (1987) Overview of biobehavioral factors in the prevention of mood disorders. In: Munoz R (ed) Depression prevention research. Hemisphere, New York

Akiskal HS, McKinney WT Jr (1975) Overview of recent research in depression: integration of ten conceptual models into a comprehensive clinical frame. Arch Gen Psychiatry 32:285–305

Akiskal HS, Djenderedjian AH, Rosenthal RH, Khani MK (1977) Cyclothymic disorder: validating criteria for inclusion in the bipolar affective group. Am J Psychiatry 134:1227–1233
Akiskal HS, Khani MK, Scott-Strauss A (1979) Cyclothymic temperamental disorders. Psychiatr Clin North Am 2:527–554
Akiskal HS, Rosenthal TL, Haykal RF, Lemmi H, Rosenthal RH, Scott-Strauss A (1980) Characterological depressions: clinical and sleep EEG findings separating "subaffective dysthymias" form "character-spectrum" disorders. Arch Gen Psychiatry 37:777–783
Akiskal HS, Hirschfeld RMA, Yerevanian BI (1983 a) The relationships of personality to affective disorders: a critical review. Arch Gen Psychiatry 40:801–810
Akiskal HS, Walker PW, Puzantian VR, King D, Rosenthal TL, Drannon M (1983 b) Bipolar outcome in the course of depressive illness. J Affective Disord 5:115–128
Akiskal HS, Lemmi H, Dickson H, King D, Yerevanian B, Van Valkenburg C (1984) Chronic depressions: Part 2. Sleep EEG differentiation of primary dysthymic disorders from anxious depressions. J Affective Disord 6:287–297
Akiskal HS, Downs J, Jordan P, Watson S, Daugherty D, Pruitt D (1985) Affective disorders in referred children and younger siblings of manic-depressives. Arch Gen Psychiatry 42:996–1003
American Psychiatric Association, Committee on Nomenclature and Statistics (1980) Diagnostic and statistical manual of mental disorders, 3rd edn. American Psychiatric Press, Washington, D. C.
Åsberg M, Schalling D, Rydin E, Traskman-Bendz L (1983) Suicide and Serotonin. In: Soubrier JP, Vedrinne J (eds) Depression and suicide. Pergamon Press, Paris
Bertelsen A, Harvald B, Hauge M (1977) A Danish study of manic-depressive disorders. Br J Psychiatry 130:338–351
Boyd J (1983) The increasing rate of suicide by firearms. N Engl J Med 308:872–874
Cassano GB, Maggini C, Akiskal HS (1983) Short-term subchronic and chronic sequelae of affective disorders. Psychiatr Clin North Am 6:55–67
Chodoff P (1972) The depressive personality: a critical review. Arch Gen Psychiatry 27:666–673
Clayton PJ (1985) Suicide. Psychiatr Clin North Am 8:203–214
DeLisio G, Maremmani I, Perugi G, Cassano GB, Deltito J, Akiskal HS (1986) Impairment of work and leisure in depressed outpatients: a preliminary communication. J Affective Disord 10:79–84
Freud S (1959) Heredity and the aetiology of the neuroses. In: Collected papers. Basic Books, New York, pp 138–154
Helgason T (1979) Epidemiological investigations concerning affective disorders. In: Schou M, Stromgren E (eds) Origin, prevention and treatment of affective disorders. Academic Press, London
Hirschfeld RM, Klerman G, Clayton P, Keller M (1983) Personality and depression: empirical findings. Arch Gen Psychiatry 40:993–998
Keller MB, Shapiro RW (1982) "Double depression": superimposition of acute depressive episodes on chronic depressive disorders. Am J Psychiatry 139:438–442
Khuri R, Akiskal HS (1983) Suicide prevention: the necessity of treating contributory psychiatric disorders. Psychiatr Clin North Am 6:193–207
Klein D, Depue R, Slater J (1985) Cyclothymia in the offspring of bipolar I and psychiatric control patients. J Abnorm Psychol 94:115–127
Kovacs M, Beck AT (1978) Maladaptive cognitive structures in depression. Am J Psychiatry 135:525–533
Kraepelin E (1921) Manic-depressive insanity and paranoia. Livingstone, Edinburgh
Kretschmer E (1936) Physique and character (E. Miller, Transl). Kegan Paul, Trench, Trubner, London
Kukopulos A, Reginaldi D, Laddomada P, Floris G, Serra G, Tondo L (1980) Course of the manic-depressive cycle and changes caused by treatments. Pharmakopsychiatr Neuro-Psychopharmakol 13:156–167

Lange J (1928) Spezieller Teil. In: Bumke O (ed) Handbook der Geisteskrankheiten. Verlag von Julius Springer, Berlin
Lewinsohn PM (1974) A behavioral approach to depression. In: Friedman RJ, Katz MM (eds) The psychology of depression: contemporary theory and research. Halstead, New York
Murphy GE (1975) The physician's responsibility for suicide I and II. Errors of commission and omission. Ann Intern Med 802:301–309
Nyman GE (1956) Variations in personality. Acta Psychiatr Scand 107:1–94
Rosenthal TL, Akiskal HS, Scott-Strauss A, Rosenthal RH, David M (1981) Familial and developmental factors in characterologic depressions. J Affective Disord 3:183–192
Schneider K (1958) Psychopathic personalities. Hamilton MW (transl) Cassell, London
Telenbach H (1980) Melancholia. Eng E (transl) Duquesne University Press, Pittsburgh

Subject Index

MIX
Papier aus verantwortungsvollen Quellen
Paper from responsible sources
FSC® C105338

If you have any concerns about our products,
you can contact us on
ProductSafety@springernature.com

In case Publisher is established outside the EU,
the EU authorized representative is:
Springer Nature Customer Service Center GmbH
Europaplatz 3, 69115 Heidelberg, Germany

Printed by Libri Plureos GmbH
in Hamburg, Germany